Paediatric Symptom Sorter

Based on an original idea by Dr Keith Hopcroft
and Dr Vincent Forte

(*Symptom Sorter*, now in its Fourth Edition (2010)
and published by Radcliffe Publishing Ltd)

Paediatric Symptom Sorter

A Sahib El-Radhi

PhD, MRCPCH, DCH

Honorary Consultant Paediatrician, Queen Mary's Hospital, Sidcup, Kent

Honorary Senior Lecturer, Medical School, London

Undergraduate and Postgraduate Examiner, Royal College of Paediatrics and

Child Health

Foreword by

James Carroll

MD

Professor of Neurology and Pediatrics

Chief, Child Neurology

Medical College of Georgia

Augusta, GA

USA

Radcliffe Publishing
London • New York

Radcliffe Publishing Ltd
33–41 Dallington Street
London
EC1V 0BB
United Kingdom

www.radcliffepublishing.com
Electronic catalogue and worldwide online ordering facility.

British Library Cataloguing in Publication Data

A catalogue record for this book is available from the British Library.

ISBN-13: 978 184619 474 0

Based on an original idea by Dr Keith Hopcroft and Dr Vincent Forte
(*Symptom Sorter*, now in its Fourth Edition (2010) and published by Radcliffe Publishing Ltd)

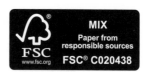
Typeset by Kate Broome, Auckland, New Zealand
Printed and bound by Hobbs the Printers, Totton, Hants, UK

CONTENTS

FOREWORD

In evaluating a child in the acute situation, it is always great to have a textbook available and to turn to the correct section of the book in a timely manner. Most textbooks, however, are treatises on diseases, mechanisms of disease, and treatment along with the theory of treatment of the disease. And so it is often not quick or easy, and time that should be spent with the child and family is consumed trying to piece together a logical approach.

Paediatric Symptom Sorter is designed to bridge the gap between the patient and the undiagnosed symptom, and to do so in a manner that is fast and felicitous to patient care. Dr El-Radhi achieves this aim by a rapid overview of the problem, a brief listing of the common and less common diagnoses, a practical differential diagnosis chart, a list of the investigations that might be necessary, and some practical advice (*Top tips* and *Red flags*). All of this is brought together in a few brief pages for each symptom.

A word about differential diagnosis: often differential diagnosis is offered merely as a listing of the possible diagnoses. Such a list does not serve to discriminate among the possibilities. Dr El-Radhi achieves this aim with a tabulation of the diagnostic possibilities versus the appropriate clinical signs and symptoms to be considered for the symptom. For example, the common causes of tremor are assessed by a consideration of family history, progressivity, and features of the examination.

The practical advice offered (*Top tips* and *Red flags*), for example the symptom of headache, is quite useful, noting here the usual lack of need for neuroimaging but the importance of looking for papilloedema.

A new book should fill a vacuum. *Paediatric Symptom Sorter* achieves the goal by a few concise, experience-based pages for almost all paediatric symptoms.

I envision that *Paediatric Symptom Sorter* will become a fixture in paediatric emergency rooms and hospital on-call rooms. I advise that the book be affixed to the furniture in a secure manner. Otherwise, it will soon disappear.

James Carroll, MD
Professor of Neurology and Pediatrics
Chief, Child Neurology
Medical College of Georgia
Augusta, GA
USA
May 2011

ABOUT THE AUTHOR

A Sahib El-Radhi, PhD, MRCPCH, DCH, completed his primary medical study at the Free University of West Berlin, Germany, where he also obtained his PhD. After working in various hospitals in Berlin, he moved to England where he worked as a paediatric Senior House Officer and Registrar. His MRCP and DCH were achieved in the 1970s. He then went to Iraq, his country of birth, to work for 5 years at a hospital on the outskirts of Baghdad. He then moved to Finland and later Kuwait as head of a paediatric department for nearly 10 years. Due to the Gulf War in 1990, he returned to Finland for two and a half years, working as a specialist paediatrician. His paediatric experience widened when he came to England in 1993 to work as a consultant paediatrician, undergraduate tutor and honorary senior lecturer, ending a long career in practising paediatrics. For over 10 years he had a leading role in managing children with enuresis in a specialist hospital clinic and outreach clinics in Bexley, Kent. He is currently serving as Honorary Consultant Paediatrician at Queen Mary's Hospital, Sidcup, Kent, and Honorary Senior Lecturer at the Medical School, London. As a guest speaker and visiting fellow, Dr El-Radhi has lectured in numerous countries worldwide at international conferences, workshops, symposia and seminars. His work as a general paediatrician in many different countries, including Germany, Finland, Iraq, Kuwait and the United Kingdom, has provided him with a wide experience of infectious and allergic diseases.

As an author over three decades, Dr El-Radhi has sat on several academic task forces and has lectured both nationally and internationally on his special interest in fever-related subjects. He has also served as an advisor and peer reviewer for several medical journals, including the *Archives of Disease in Childhood*. He has published over 30 papers in indexed journals and editorials, as well as having contributed to several paediatric books. Dr El-Radhi has spent most of his medical career in research performing numerous controlled and multi-centre studies. He has been privileged to be an undergraduate and postgraduate examiner for the Royal College of Paediatrics and Child Health, and in particular the MRCPCH and DCH exams, for over 10 years.

LIST OF ABBREVIATIONS

A&E	accident and emergency		CRF	chronic renal failure
ACS	acute confusional state		CRP	c-reactive protein
AD	atopic dermatitis		CSF	cerebrospinal fluid
ADH	antidiuretic hormone		CT	computed tomography
AED	antiepileptic drug		CTD	connective tissue disease
AHG	acute herpetic gingivostomatitis		CULLP	congenital unilateral lower lip palsy
ANA	anti-nuclear antibodies		CVS	congenital varicella syndrome
AOS	arterial oxygen saturation		DHEAS	dehydroepiandrosterone sulfate
AR	allergic rhinitis		DI	diabetes insipidus
ARF	acute renal failure		DIC	disseminated intravascular coagulation
ASO	antistreptolysin			
BC	blood culture		DKA	diabetic ketoacidosis
BG	blood glucose		DM	diabetes mellitus
BPV	benign paroxysmal vertigo		DP	delayed puberty
CAH	congenital adrenal hyperplasia		EBV	Epstein–Barr virus
CANOMAD	chronic ataxic neuropathy with ophthalmoplegia, M-protein, agglutination, and disialosyl antibodies		ECG	electrocardiogram
			EEG	electroencephalogram
			EKC	epidemic keratoconjunctivitis
			EM	erythema multiforme
CCF	congestive cardiac failure		EMLA	eutectic mixture of local anaesthetics
CCMT	congenital cutis marmorata telangiectatica		ENT	ear, nose and throat
CD	Crohn's disease		EOAE	evoked otoacoustic emissions
CF	cystic fibrosis		ESR	erythrocyte sedimentation rate
CFS	chronic fatigue syndrome			
CHARGE	coloboma, heart defect, atresia of the choanae, retarded growth, genital hypoplasia and ear anomaly		FB	foreign body
			FBC	full blood count
			MFBC	maximal functional bladder capacity
CHD	congenital heart disease		FCUS	familial cold urticaria syndrome
CMV	cytomegalovirus			
CNS	central nervous system		FMF	familial Mediterranean fever
CPK	creatine phosphokinase		FS	febrile seizures
CREST	calcinosis, Raynaud's phenomenon, oesophageal dysmotility, sclerodactyly and telangiectasia		FSH	follicle-stimulating hormone
			FTT	failure to thrive
			FWF	fever without focus

GAHS	group A β-haemolytic streptococci	
GE	gastroenteritis	
GF	glandular fever	
GH	growth hormone	
GI	gastrointestinal	
GN	glomerulonephritis	
GnRH	gonadotropins-releasing hormone	
GO	gastro-oesophageal	
HAV	hepatitis A virus	
Hb	haemoglobin	
HbA2	haemoglobin alpha 2	
HbF	haemoglobin F	
HbS	haemoglobin S	
HD	Hirschsprung's disease	
HL	Hodgkin's lymphoma	
HHT	hereditary haemorrhagic telangiectasia	
HHV-6	human herpesvirus 6	
HIDS	hyperimmunoglobuliaemia D syndrome	
HIE	hypoxic-ischaemic encephalopathy	
HIV	human immunodeficiency virus	
HSP	Henöch–Schönlein purpura	
HUS	haemolytic-uraemic syndrome	
HVA	homovanillic acid	
IBD	inflammatory bowel disease	
IBS	irritable bowel syndrome	
ICP	intracranial pressure	
ID	intellectual disability	
IDA	iron-deficiency anaemia	
IgM-RF	immunoglobulin M rheumatoid factor	
IH	inguinal hernia	
IQ	intelligence quotient	
ISO	idiopathic scrotal oedema	
ITP	idiopathic thrombocytopenic purpura	
IV	intravenous	
JHR	Jarisch–Herxheimer reaction	
JRA	juvenile rheumatoid arthritis	
KLS	Kleine–Levin syndrome	
LAMB	A syndrome of lentigines, atrial myxoma, mucocutaneous myxoma and blue nevi	
LEOPARD	A syndrome of lentigines, ECG abnormalities, ocular hypertelorism, pulmonary stenosis, abnormal genitalia, retarded growth, deafness	
LFT	liver function tests	
LH	luteinising hormone	
LMN	lower motor neurone	
LP	lumbar puncture	
LRTI	lower respiratory tract infection	
MCV	mean cell volume	
MELAS	mitochondrial encephalopathy, lactic acidosis and stroke-like episodes	
MRI	magnetic resonance imaging	
MSPS	musculoskeletal pain syndrome	
MWS	Muckle–Wells syndrome	
NAI	non-accidental injury	
NCSE	non-convulsive status epilepticus	
NE	nocturnal enuresis	
NF-1	neurofibromatosis type 1	
NFLE	nocturnal frontal lobe epilepsy	
NIDDM	non-insulin-dependent diabetes mellitus	
NMD	neuromuscular disorders	
NS	nephrotic syndrome	
NSAID	non-steroidal anti-inflammatory drug	
NUG	necrotising ulcerative gingivostomatitis	
NV	neonatal varicella	
OCD	obsessive–compulsive disorder	
OE	otitis externa	
OM	otitis media	
OME	otitis media with effusion	
OSAS	obstructive sleep apnoea syndrome	
POS	polycystic ovary syndrome	
PCR	polymerase chain reaction	
PF	periodic fever	

PFAPA	periodic fever/aphthous stomatitis/pharyngitis/ cervical adenitis	ROP	retinopathy of prematurity
		RP	rectal prolapse
		RTA	renal tubular acidosis
PHACE	a syndrome of posterior fossa, haemangioma, arterial, cardiac and eye abnormalities	SA	septic arthritis
		SCA	sickle-cell anaemia
		SCBU	special care baby unit
PHN	post-herpetic neuralgia	SD	seborrhoeic dermatitis
PID	pelvic inflammatory disease	SE	status epilepticus
PIH	post-inflammatory hyperpigmentation	SLE	systemic lupus erythematosus
		SNE	secondary nocturnal enuresis
PLMD	periodic limb movement disorder	SS	short stature
PNE	primary nocturnal enuresis	STD	sexually transmitted disease
POS	polycystic ovarian syndrome	SVT	supraventricular tachycardia
PP	precocious puberty	TB	tuberculosis
PPP	partial precocious puberty	TDC	thyroglossal duct cyst
PS	pyloric stenosis	TFT	thyroid function test
PSGN	poststreptococcal glomerulonephritis	TORCH	toxoplasmosis, rubella, cytomegalovirus and herpes
PT	prothrombin time	TRAPS	TNF-receptor associated periodic syndrome
PTT	partial thromboplastin time		
PUO	pyrexia of unknown origin	TV	television
RAP	recurrent abdominal pain	U&E	urea and electrolytes
RAST	radioallergosorbent test	UMN	upper motor neurone
RBC	red blood cell	URTI	upper respiratory tract infection
RBC/hpf	red blood cells per high-power field		
		UTI	urinary tract infection
RDS	respiratory distress syndrome	VD	vaginal discharge
RE	rectal examination	VMA	vanillylmandelic acid
ReA	reactive arthritis	VN	vestibular neuritis
RF	rheumatic fever	VR	vasomotor rhinitis
ReF	relapsing fever	VT	ventricular tachycardia
RFT	renal function tests	WBC	white blood cell count
RhF	rheumatoid factor	WPW	Wolff–Parkinson–White

INTRODUCTION

When I reached an agreement with Radcliffe Publishing to write this book I was full of enthusiasm, knowing how important the subject of differential diagnosis is in paediatrics and recognising the lack of books on the subject. I was, however, not fully aware of the difficulties in preparing and writing such a book. The first problem arose when I needed to choose which possible diagnoses should be labelled *Common* and which should be labelled *Rare*, and which ones should appear under *Infants* and which under *Children*. Although it was easy to put the majority of diagnoses under the appropriate heading, for others the distinction was not so clear. When it comes to the heading, *Differential diagnosis at a glance*, some paediatricians may select *Possible* for *Yes* or *No*, or *Yes* for *Possible* or *No*. Under *Recommended investigations* experienced paediatricians may recommend fewer or more tests for the subject addressed. Under *Top tips* and *Red flags*, some comments appearing under one heading may be more appropriately placed under the other. While I accept the criticism from my colleagues that some of these selections may be wrong and considered mistakes, my response is that these could reflect normal different views that are often found among paediatricians. It is commonly accepted in paediatric practice that there are grey areas without clear-cut distinguishing features and there is no right or wrong in many subjects. It is hoped that accuracy and scientific evidence have prevailed in every section of the book, which came as a result of long personal paediatric experience and repeated revision, backed by a thorough search of the literature. Diagnosis is based on the best available evidence and established guidelines have been included wherever available and appropriate.

The vast majority of paediatric books on the market are system-based. Children, however, present with a plethora of symptoms and to reach the right diagnosis from these symptoms, clinicians often have to work through a differential diagnosis to solve a clinical problem. It is hoped that this book will aid the clinician in reaching the correct diagnosis easily and quickly. This symptom-based book has been written for all professionals who deal with sick children, including junior and senior paediatricians, primary care doctors and, particularly, those who need rapid reference, e.g. doctors on call. Paediatric nurses, with their increasing role in managing sick children, may use the book as a reference in their clinical activity. Medical students, when on paediatric wards or in A&E departments as part of their attachment, may also use differential diagnosis for discussion with their qualified colleagues.

Each symptom is analysed as follows.

The clinician overview

This contains an introduction to the subject in preparation for what is to follow. As an overview this section can be seen as an abstract of the whole symptom. A definition of the subject is included whenever appropriate.

Possible diagnoses

This lists many possible diagnoses, five of which are considered common, with an onset in infants (below the age of 1 year) and in older children; the remaining diagnoses are considered rare. Due to space restrictions, there is no discussion or further elaboration in the vast majority of these rare diagnoses. The reader, however, can turn to the literature to obtain more knowledge on the subject.

Differential diagnosis at a glance

This section provides differential diagnosis of the five common diagnoses listed in the previous section. As the title indicates, it offers a quick guide to key features used to differentiate each diagnosis from the other four.

Recommended investigations

This section provides a list of investigations that should assist the clinician in establishing the diagnosis. Simple investigations, such as urine and FBC, top the list, followed by more sophisticated tests such as MRI or invasive techniques such as biopsy.

Each investigation is given an asterisk rating between * and *** to indicate importance; an investigation showing three asterisks, for example, is more strongly recommended than an investigation with one asterisk.

TOP TIPS

This offers tips and hints to lead the clinician to reach the correct diagnosis. It also contains general knowledge related to the subject discussed.

This section provides a list of warning signs to ensure clinicians do not miss or neglect certain aspects of the presentation. Such errors may lead to increased morbidity and possible fatality.

How to use this book

Symptoms occurring in children are too numerous to be included in any book addressing the subject of 'differential diagnosis'. However, most symptoms, including common ones, have been enlisted. The book is arranged in sections, where each section corresponds to an anatomical region, e.g. Oral, Abdomen, etc. The Abdomen section, for example, contains symptoms related to abdominal diseases, e.g. abdominal pain, diarrhoea, vomiting and jaundice. These are discussed first in the book while diseases of the urinary tract are discussed at the end. However, not all symptoms presented originate in the corresponding anatomical region, e.g. pain felt in the abdomen may originate in the spine or chest. The reader will easily find all causes of the abdominal pain symptom, irrespective of its origin, practically divided into five *Common* and *Rare* causes, with *Infants* and *Children* subsets. As most causes of the symptom originate in the anatomical region, e.g. in the abdomen, the reader is advised to focus on them first, and then move on to other causes outside the region for expansion of the differential diagnosis if the presenting symptom does not appear to belong within the region.

The *Paediatric Symptom Sorter* is quick and easy to use and designed as a rapid reference. Occasionally some symptoms are repeatedly discussed, e.g. Henöch–Schönlein purpura (HSP) appears in abdominal pain, skin purpura and penile swelling. Therefore, some information is repeated. This is not only inevitable in providing better understanding and a complete overview of the subject under discussion but also necessary for the reader, who will refer to the section to obtain the information required to lead them to the correct diagnosis. It also avoids referring readers to other sections in order to complete the information. Any such cross-references have been kept to a minimum.

The author recommends that the book is kept readily available for use whenever possible during on-call duties, such as in A&E, to retrieve relevant information in a speedy way. Unless the case presents as an emergency, professionals should have time to read through the differential diagnosis in case the symptom presented is not a straightforward one and a differential diagnosis is required. It is more important to come up with a correct diagnosis to the case, even if slightly delayed, rather than a hasty diagnosis that is incorrect.

A question may arise about the need for such a book. Medical students receive little or no teaching about differential diagnoses. Lectures addressing the subject are few or non-existent and books on the subject are hard to come by. These reasons provided the impetus to write this book. This is the first edition and I feel the market will eagerly receive it. I do hope that it will become a popular and essential guide, read by many of my fellow paediatricians. Their comments and feedback will be important in the preparation of future editions of the *Paediatric Symptom Sorter*.

A Sahib El-Radhi
May 2011

Abdomen

Acute abdominal pain

Chronic/recurrent abdominal pain

Abdominal distension

Vomiting

Vomiting blood (haematemesis)

Gastrointestinal bleeding (rectal bleeding)

Diarrhoea

Constipation

Jaundice

ACUTE ABDOMINAL PAIN

The clinician overview

Acute abdominal pain is a common complaint seen in the A&E department. The main objective in dealing with a child with abdominal pain is to differentiate between benign and self-limited conditions, such as constipation or gastroenteritis (GE), and more life-threatening surgical conditions, such as volvulus or appendicitis. The term 'acute abdomen' refers to an intra-abdominal condition that usually requires a surgical intervention. Pain originating from the liver, pancreas and upper intestine is typically felt in the epigastric area; pain originating from the small intestine or appendiceal inflammation is felt typically in the periumbilical area (because the pathway is at the T10 level); and pain from the distal colon and urinary tract is felt in the suprapubic area. Extra-abdominal conditions, such as pneumonia or pharyngitis, are important causes of abdominal pain.

Possible diagnoses

INFANTS
Common
- Hunger
- Infection elsewhere (e.g. ear)
- Oesophagitis (GO reflux)
- Gastroenteritis (GE)
- Evening colic

Rare
- Incarcerated hernia
- Intussusception, volvulus
- Intestinal obstruction
- Urinary tract infection (UTI)

CHILDREN
- Gastroenteritis (GE)
- Psychogenic (e.g. anxiety, school phobia)
- UTI
- Appendicitis
- Mesenteric adenitis

- Referred pain (e.g. pneumonia, pharyngitis)
- Constipation
- Renal stones
- Pancreatitis
- Oesophagitis (GO reflux)
- Hepatitis
- Intussusception
- Intestinal obstruction
- Crohn's disease
- Diabetic ketoacidosis (DKA)
- Sickle-cell anaemia

◪ Gilbert's syndrome
◪ Gallstones

Differential diagnosis at a glance

	GE	Psychogenic	UTI	Appendicitis	Mesenteric adenitis
With diarrhoea	Yes	No	Possible	Possible	No
Diffuse pain location	Yes	Yes	No	No	Possible
Abdominal tenderness	Possible	Possible	Possible	Yes	Yes
Localised pain	No	No	Yes	Yes	Possible
With fever	Possible	No	Yes	Yes	Yes

Recommended investigations

***   Urinalysis with urine culture to confirm UTI. Dipsticks: the presence of positive nitrate and leukocytes suggests the diagnosis; their absence makes the diagnosis very unlikely.

***   Stool culture for bacterial GE; viral antigen detection for rotavirus.

***   FBC: leukocytosis suggests inflammatory causes, marked leukocytosis (leukomoid reaction) seen occasionally in pneumonia.

***   LFT to diagnose hepatitis; blood glucose, U&E and blood gases to rule out DKA in case of associated vomiting with a history of polydipsia and polyuria.

**   Abdomen X-ray may show signs of impacted stool in constipation or signs of intestinal obstruction.

***   Abdominal ultrasound scan for suspected cases of renal stones or gallstones.

TOP TIPS

◪ Abdominal examination should be performed with extreme gentleness and compassion; careful hands-off inspection being the first step, followed by a non-intimidating position of sitting down or kneeling to be at the same level as the child. A young child is best examined in a parent's arms or lap. Distracting the child while palpating the abdomen is very helpful.

◪ It is worth asking the child to point with their finger to the area 'where it hurts most'.

◪ A student or a postgraduate doctor in an examination who hurts the child while examining the abdomen should expect a failure mark as a result.

◪ Remember, the closer the pain to the umbilicus the less likely it is to be of organic disease.

◪ The primary objective of managing a child with acute abdominal pain is to exclude a surgical condition.

- A thorough extra-abdominal examination is indicated as the cause of the pain could well be in the throat, lung, spine or hips (e.g. synovitis).
- Remember that the typical abdomen in GE is non-distended, soft and mildly tender but with little or no guarding.
- The use of a sedative or analgesic does not increase the risk of misdiagnosis.
- Urinalysis is essential in every child with abdominal pain and fever, particularly if the fever has no localised source.
- Beware that GE can present with abdominal pain only prior to developing diarrhoea.
- When a diagnosis of mesenteric adenitis is made, stool culture for the bacteria yersinia should be performed.
- It is the clinician's skill to differentiate between a self-limited process (e.g. viral GE, constipation) and more life-threatening surgical emergencies (e.g. intussusception).
- Extra-abdominal examination is important as tonsillitis and lower-lobe pneumonia can produce abdominal pain and mimic abdominal emergencies, e.g. appendicitis. Thorough examination of these sites is essential.

Red flags

- Beware that GE may mask appendicitis, and abdominal pain in DKA may mimic appendicitis.
- An acute abdominal pain that makes the child miserable and uncooperative is serious and often requires surgical intervention.
- Perforation of the appendix presents as an acute abdomen. Children typically have a longer history of pain, greater systemic effect, high fever, more generalised tenderness and minimal or absent bowel sounds.
- A young child with mild abdominal pain, vomiting and clinical signs of dehydration but no ketones in the urine should be suspected of having an inborn error of metabolism.

NOTES:

CHRONIC/RECURRENT ABDOMINAL PAIN

The clinician overview

Recurrent abdominal pain (RAP) is a very common symptom estimated to affect around 10% of school-age children. The symptom is significant because it is responsible for a high rate of morbidity, missed school days, high use of health resources and parental anxiety. RAP is defined as pain severe enough to interfere with activity, with intermittent and at least three recurrent episodes occurring over a 3-month period (Apley's criteria). In 1958 Apley estimated that only 8% of patients with RAP had, after extensive investigations, organic pathology. Nowadays a higher estimate is accepted, mainly because irritable bowel syndrome (IBS) has been recognised as an important cause of RAP and a high rate of detecting pathology by the recent imaging technology. Parasites, such as giardia, are a common and important cause of RAP in developing countries. Most children with RAP have no organic diseases (functional abdominal pain) and present typically as a central abdominal pain, with no guarding, rebound or rigidity, and without abnormal physical sign on investigation. Recurrent crying episodes in an infant who draws their legs up and appears to be in pain are defined as colic, not RAP.

Possible diagnoses

INFANTS
Common
- Infantile colic (evening colic)
- GO reflux
- Lactose intolerance
- Cow's milk protein allergy
- Parasites (e.g. giardia)

Rare
- Coeliac disease
- Meckel's diverticulum
- Child abuse
- Scurvy

CHILDREN

- Functional RAP (psychogenic, e.g. school phobia)
- Food intolerance/allergy
- Abdominal migraine (and migraine variant of cyclic vomiting)
- IBS
- Parasites (e.g. giardia)

- Inflammatory bowel disease (IBD, e.g. Crohn's disease, ulcerative colitis)
- Recurrent urinary tract infection (UTI)
- Gilbert's syndrome
- Familial Mediterranean fever
- Porphyria

- ☑ Sickle-cell anaemia (SCA)
- ☑ Coeliac disease
- ☑ Meckel's diverticulum
- ☑ Pancreatitis
- ☑ Hepatitis
- ☑ Stones in the urinary system and gall bladder
- ☑ Peptic ulcer
- ☑ Lead poisoning

Differential diagnosis at a glance

	Functional RAP	Food intolerance	Abdominal migraine	IBS	Parasites
Weight loss	No	Possible	No	Possible	Possible
Bloody diarrhoea	No	Possible	No	No	No
Stool changes	No	Yes	No	Yes	Yes
Vomiting	No	Possible	Possible	No	Possible
Associated malabsorption	No	Possible	No	No	Possible

Recommended investigations

*** Dipsticks: haematuria may suggest renal stones; leukocytes and nitrite UTI.

*** Stool for parasites and culture.

*** FBC with CRP: useful in suggesting inflammation and infection; anaemia in SCA.

*** Blood for LFT to diagnose hepatitis, Gilbert's disease.

*** Coeliac screening tests in blood.

*** Screen testing in stool for *Helicobacter pylori*.

*** Abdominal ultrasound scan: will confirm renal stones or gallstones.

** Endoscopy: in case of high suspicion of an organic cause.

TOP TIPS

- The history should provide the basis for diagnosis and investigation. The vast majority of diagnoses are made by careful history, thorough examination and minimal investigation.
- The closer the pain is to the umbilicus, the less likely it is to be significant. Pain away from the umbilicus is suggestive of an organic cause.
- Extra-abdominal causes of abdominal pain are common in children, and they can even dominate the clinical picture. Examples are acute tonsillitis, lower-lobe pneumonia and testicular disease.
- Functional abdominal diseases are suggested by symptom-free intervals, healthy appearance of the child and absence of abnormalities on examination; organic diseases tend to have chronic or progressive course and presence of abnormalities on examination.
- Psychogenic causes of RAP should be diagnosed on positive grounds, not simply by excluding organic disease.
- Children of a parent with gastrointestinal disease are more likely to have RAP.
- If a child's RAP is thought to have psychogenic cause, it is not good practice to tell the parents 'the cause is psychological'. Offering support and reassurance that their child is healthy and the abdominal pain will not affect the child's well-being is of great comfort to the parents.
- Pain in constipation is often overrated as a diagnostic entity. It should not be made simply because no other cause except constipation is elicited from the history and examination.
- Note that food intolerance/allergy is the second-most-common cause (after psychogenic cause) of RAP in an otherwise healthy child. Eliminating the suspected food item (particularly milk or wheat) for about 2 weeks is the best diagnostic and therapeutic tool. Blood or skin testing is of limited value.

Red flags

- An underlying organic cause for RAP is suggested if the pain is in the flanks, suprapubic area, persistently in the right or left upper or lower quadrant, or associated with vomiting, diarrhoea or fever.
- Beware that a child known to have recurrent functional abdominal pain could present one day with an organic cause that may need surgical intervention.
- Always ask whether the pain was followed, not preceded, by vomiting, as this is suggestive of appendicitis.
- Remember that often the frequency of RAP is greater and the duration of symptoms longer in children who have been victims of sexual abuse. If such a case is suspected, the child should be protected in a hospital environment until the conclusive diagnosis is made.

NOTES:

ABDOMINAL DISTENSION

The clinician overview

Abdominal distension is defined as an increase girth of the abdomen caused by air, fluid, stool, mass or organomegaly. It is a common clinical finding, particularly in neonates, and must be evaluated carefully. A long history of abdominal distension associated with loose motions and being underweight is very suggestive of malabsorption, and disacharidase deficiency and coeliac disease are the most common causes. Mild abdominal distension in a thriving and well toddler is very common and normal. Vomiting, particularly bile-stained, suggests intestinal obstruction. Other rare but important causes of abdominal distension in infants and toddlers include neuroblastoma and nephroblastoma.

Possible diagnoses

INFANTS
Common
- Mechanical ventilation
- Sepsis
- Intestinal atresia or stenosis
- Meconium plug or ileus, necrotising enterocolitis
- Abdominal mass (tumour, hepatosplenomegaly)

Rare
- Renal vein thrombosis (flank mass)
- Hepatomegaly, splenomegaly
- Tumour (nephroblastoma, neuroblastoma)
- Imperforate hymen
- Hydrometrocolpos
- Gartner's duct cyst
- Prolapsed ureterocele, urethrocele
- Chloramphenicol toxicity (grey syndrome)
- Colonic atresia, stenosis, imperforate anus

CHILDREN
- Physiological in toddlers (usually mild)
- Malabsorption (coeliac disease, CF, giardia)
- Intestinal obstruction
- Constipation
- Abdominal mass (e.g. neuroblastoma)

- Glycogen storage disease
- Hirschsprung's disease
- Ascites (e.g. nephrotic syndrome)
- Ovarian cyst
- Kwashiorkor (in the tropics)

Differential diagnosis at a glance

	Physiological in toddlers	Malabsorption	Intestinal obstruction	Constipation	Abdominal mass
Thriving	Yes	No	Possible	Yes	Possible
Diarrhoea	No	Possible	No	No	No
Palpable mass	No	No	Possible	Yes	Yes
Failure to thrive	No	Yes	No	No	Possible
Vomiting	No	Possible	Yes	No	Possible

Recommended investigations

Investigation is determined by the history and clinical findings.

*** Urine for VMA and HVA in suspected cases of neuroblastoma.

*** FBC, CRP and culture to screen for infection. BC to rule out sepsis, tests for coeliac disease.

*** Plasma protein, albumin, U&E for suspected malabsorption and malnutrition or ascites.

*** Stool microscopy for giardia, pus cells, fat droplets, clinitest tab for reducible substance and culture.

*** Plain chest and abdominal X-ray for intestinal obstruction, detecting of tumour, calcification in nephroblastoma and detection of faecal masses in severe constipation.

*** Ultrasound scan to confirm intra-abdominal tumour, renal pathology or ovarian cyst.

*** Barium enema may suggest Hirschsprung's disease; rectal biopsy confirms it.

*** CT or MRI to evaluate abdominal masses and determine their relationship to other organs.

*** Sweat test for cystic fibrosis (CF).

*** Bone scan to detect possible metastasis in neuroblastoma.

TOP TIPS

▱ History is of paramount importance in giving a diagnostic clue: duration of the distension (acute or chronic), any weight loss, diarrhoea or vomiting; is the vomiting bile-stained?

▱ In the absence of an intestinal obstruction, repeated vomiting causes bilious vomiting through refluxed duodenal contents into the stomach. Otherwise, bilious vomiting usually indicates obstruction below the second part of the duodenum.

▱ A child who has failed to thrive with abdominal distension should not be considered physiologic; is very likely to have malabsorption.

▱ In malabsorption and malnutrition, initial weight loss is typical; when the disease becomes chronic, deceleration in height ensues.

▱ Although hydronephrosis and multicystic dysplastic kidney are the two most common abdominal masses, they rarely cause abdominal distension.

- A lower intestinal obstruction (e.g. Hirschsprung's disease) usually presents with abdominal distension and late vomiting, while an upper one presents with early vomiting and no distension.
- Causes of abdominal distension in the tropics differ from those in developed countries; parasites (e.g. giardia, worms) and kwashiorkor usually prevail in the tropics.
- Beware of two important causes of chronic distension: malabsorption and coeliac disease.

Red flags

- All children with intestinal obstruction should receive a nasogastric suction catheter; failure to decompress the stomach could lead to gastric rupture, aspiration or respiratory distress secondary to diaphragmatic compression.
- Excluding toddler physiological abdominal distension, abdominal distension should always be considered serious requiring usually urgent investigation.
- Priority remains to exclude life-threatening surgical causes of abdominal distension such as intestinal obstruction.

NOTES:

VOMITING

The clinician overview

Vomiting is a forceful action accomplished by a downward contraction of the diaphragm along with tightening of the abdominal muscles against an open sphincter propelling gastric contents out. Retching signals the beginning of vomiting. These steps are coordinated by the medullary vomiting centre, which receives afferent signals from the gastrointestinal tract, the blood stream, equilibrium system of the inner ear and central nervous system (CNS). Because vomiting is a very common symptom in children, it should be evaluated in the clinical context with other associated symptoms. The clinician should be in a position to determine the degree of seriousness of vomiting. This section only discusses vomiting as a major symptom. Unlike vomiting, which is a forceful action, regurgitation indicates a discharge of gastric contents without effort and nausea.

Possible diagnoses

INFANTS

Common
- ☑ GO reflux
- ☑ Swallowed blood or fluid during delivery
- ☑ Systemic infection
- ☑ Intestinal obstruction (e.g. necrotising enterocolitis)
- ☑ Pyloric stenosis (PS)

Rare
- ☑ Overfeeding (mainly in premature baby)
- ☑ Sepsis
- ☑ Milk protein/lactose intolerance
- ☑ Inborn errors of metabolism (e.g. galactosaemia)
- ☑ Rumination
- ☑ Oesophageal atresia
- ☑ Intussusception
- ☑ Subdural haematoma

CHILDREN

- ☑ Gastroenteritis
- ☑ Systemic infection (e.g. pneumonia, urinary tract infection)
- ☑ GO reflux
- ☑ Migraine
- ☑ Medication (e.g. antipyretics, antibiotics)

- ☑ Appendicitis
- ☑ Meningitis
- ☑ Pregnancy
- ☑ Periodic syndrome (cyclic vomiting)
- ☑ Intestinal obstruction
- ☑ Increased intracranial pressure (e.g. tumour)
- ☑ Pertussis
- ☑ Inflammatory bowel disease
- ☑ Peptic ulcer
- ☑ Norovirus

◪ Pancreatitis
◪ Inborn errors of metabolism
◪ Renal or biliary colic
◪ Chemotherapy

Differential diagnosis at a glance

	Gastroenteritis	Systemic infection	GO reflux	Migraine	Medication
Diarrhoea	Yes	Possible	No	No	Possible
Associated dehydration	Yes	Possible	No	No	Possible
Thriving	Possible	Yes	Possible	Yes	Yes
Fever	Possible	Yes	No	No	No
Acute history	Yes	Yes	No	Yes	Yes

Recommended investigations

Investigation should be directed according to the history and clinical findings. These can suggest a diagnosis in the majority of cases, e.g. gastroenteritis, medication or PS.

***   Urine for reducing substance to diagnose galactosaemia; blood gases, amino acids and other metabolic screen tests are required for inborn error of metabolism.

**   Blood for FBC, CRP, U&E for more persistent vomiting; leukocytosis and high CRP suggest bacterial infection (e.g. sepsis, pneumonia).

**   Stool for microscopy and culture for significant gastroenteritis.

***   Abdominal and chest X-ray is useful in intestinal obstruction.

**   Abdominal ultrasound scan may confirm PS.

TOP TIPS

◪ About 50% of neonates and infants regurgitate or vomit several times a day after feeding. If they are otherwise well and thriving and the vomit looks like feeds, a diagnosis of GO reflux can be made.

◪ Most infants with GO reflux do well aged 6–12 months; rare complications include oesophagitis, aspiration pneumonia and abnormal neck and head posturing (Sandifer's syndrome).

◪ PS is differentiated from GO reflux by vomiting (projectile), occurring in the first 2–3 weeks of life in a baby who is hungry, with visible gastric peristalsis and a palpation of an 'olive' in the right upper quadrant. With reflux, children vomit during or immediately after feeding.

- A palpable pyloric tumour (present in about 50% of cases) is pathognomonic for PS. An ultrasound is a very useful tool in experienced hands; a thickness of > 4 mm suggests the diagnosis.
- Cyclic vomiting is characterised by frequent episodic vomiting with symptom-free intervals. Family history of migraine supports the diagnosis. An inborn error of metabolism needs to be excluded.
- Anti-emetics, analogue antidiarrhoeal drugs, are rarely used in paediatrics. Finding out the underlying cause of the vomiting is far more important than spending time looking up anti-emetics in the British National Formulary. Exceptions are for chemotherapy and occasionally migraine-induced vomiting.

Red flags

- Consider inborn errors of metabolism in the differential diagnosis of any severely ill neonate who presents with poor feeding, lethargy, vomiting and convulsion in early life. The condition is often lethal unless prompt treatment is initiated.
- Although dehydration is the main complication of vomiting, particularly in infants and young children, hypochloraemic hypokalaemic alkalosis or bleeding from tears in the distal oesophagus may sometimes be complications as well.
- Beware that although bilious vomiting occasionally occurs after severe vomiting and retching, it usually suggests intestinal obstruction requiring immediate medical attention.
- Beware that pain usually precedes vomiting in appendicitis and intestinal obstruction.
- Not all vomiting with headache is migraine; a CNS lesion such as a brain tumour must be excluded.
- Vomiting usually causes metabolic alkalosis. The presence of metabolic acidosis is suggestive of gastroenteritis or an inborn error of metabolism. The latter possibility is high on the list in the presence of metabolic acidosis without diarrhoea.

NOTES:

VOMITING BLOOD (HAEMATEMESIS)

The clinician overview

Gastrointestinal (GI) bleeding may originate anywhere from the mouth to the anus. It is much less common in children than in adults because of the rarity of GI cancers. Haematemesis, with or without melaena, usually indicates a bleed from a site proximal to the ligament of Treitz of the duodenum (proximal GI tract). Haematochezia refers to a distal bleeding. When haematemesis is caused by brisk bleeding it usually indicates an arterial source, while coffee ground emesis results from bleeding that has slowed or stopped, or from conversion of the red colour of Hb to brown haematin by gastric acid. The causes of haematemesis vary according to the age of the child and whether there are other associated symptoms. Haematemesis (usually associated with nausea, vomiting, pain and possible tenderness of the abdomen) must be differentiated from haemoptysis (associated with cough, a frothy colour, crackle noises on lung auscultation and evidence of pulmonary disease) and swallowed epistaxis (blood present in the nose, dripping into the posterior nasopharynx).

Possible diagnoses

INFANTS
Common
- Swallowed maternal blood (during birth)
- Swallowed blood from cracked nipple during breastfeeding
- Oesophagitis secondary to GO reflux
- Necrotising enterocolitis
- Thrombocytopenia

Rare
- Coagulation disorder
- Disseminated intravascular coagulation
- Meckel's diverticulum
- Haemophilia

CHILDREN
- Drugs (non-steroidal anti-inflammatory drugs (NSAIDs))
- Gastritis
- Mallory–Weiss syndrome
- Oesophagitis (GO reflux)
- Swallowed blood (e.g. epistaxis)

- Oesophageal varices (usually large haematemesis)
- Gastric erosion or ulcer
- Thrombocytopenia
- Swallowing of foreign body
- Haemophilia
- Gastric tumour

Differential diagnosis at a glance

	Drugs	Gastritis	M–W syndrome	Oesophagitis	Swallowed blood
Associated pain	Possible	Yes	Possible	Yes	No
Preceded by vomiting	Possible	Possible	Yes	Yes	No
Prior severe retching	No	No	Yes	No	No
Massive bleeding	Possible	Possible	Yes	No	No
Occurrence in infancy	Possible	Possible	No	Yes	No

Recommended investigations

***   FBC: anaemia suggests chronic blood loss or large vomiting of blood; thrombocytopenia suggests a haematological cause of the haematemesis.

***   Coagulation studies (PT, PTT, clotting factors, LFT) for bleeding or coagulation disease.

***   Apt test will determine if the haematemesis is maternal (blood denatures with alkali) or fetal (blood does not denature with alkali) in origin.

***   Abdomen plain radiographs useful for detecting necrotising enterocolitis, foreign body.

***   Abdominal ultrasound scan is the first line of imaging for suspected intussusception; if confirmed, an enema is used for reduction.

**   Endoscopy for upper GI bleed.

TOP TIPS

- Mallory–Weiss tear, described in 1929 in association with alcohol bingeing, is rare in children. GO reflux remains one of the most common causes.
- In the majority of cases of haematemesis the history will suggest the likely diagnosis and tests required.
- The most common cause of haematemesis in a well full-term baby is swallowing of maternal blood during delivery or from the breast. Inspection of the mother's breast or expressed milk will suggest the diagnosis. Diagnosis can be confirmed with an Apt test performed on blood aspirated from the stomach.
- Vomiting blood may be bright red or dark resembling coffee grounds; the latter indicates digestion of blood by gastric juice.
- Haematemesis is always a frightening experience for parents. There should be a low threshold to admit the child; this alone would relieve the parents' anxiety.
- Haematemesis caused by medications, particularly NSAIDs, is under-reported and underestimated; it is always worth taking a detailed history of the recent intake of drugs.
- When a child has haematemesis while taking NSAIDs, the haematemesis is more likely the result of the drugs rather than 'viral gastritis'.

◪ Although precise diagnosis is important, resuscitation and stabilisation of the child and possible blood transfusion is essential before any diagnostic investigation.

◪ Aspirin should not be given to children (except in certain indications, e.g. Kawasaki's disease). Parents may not be aware that many over-the-counter cough remedies and analgesics contain aspirin.

◪ A Mallory–Weiss tear (linear laceration at the gastro-oesophageal junction) may occur after a single episode of vomiting. Children with portal hypertension or hepatic insufficiency have a high risk of developing this tear.

NOTES:

GASTROINTESTINAL BLEEDING (RECTAL BLEEDING)

The clinician overview

Gastrointestinal (GI) bleeding is a fairly common, anxiety-provoking complaint. Massive bleeding is, however, rare. Damage to the GI mucosa is the most common cause of bleeding, with the exception of small intestinal mucosa. This part of the intestine is the least likely cause of bleeding. Beyond the neonatal period, anal fissures are the most common cause of rectal bleeding. The child presents with painful defecation and small blood streaks on the surface of the stool. Haematochezia, passage of bright-red blood, usually indicates a bleed from a site below the ligament of Treitz of the duodenum, i.e. blood has not been in contact with gastric juice. Bright blood mixed with loose stools suggests a bleeding site above the rectum (colitis, e.g. infectious or ulcerative colitis). Melaena, the passage of black tarry stools, usually indicates an acute upper GI bleed.

Possible diagnoses

INFANTS
Common
- Any cause of haematemesis
- Swallowed maternal blood
- Vitamin K deficiency
- Necrotising enterocolitis
- Anal fissure

Rare
- Intussusception
- Thrombocytopenia
- Volvulus
- Milk protein intolerance
- Drugs
- Neonatal stress ulcer
- Polyp
- Haemorrhagic disease
- Intestinal haemangioma
- Haemangiomas

CHILDREN
- Any cause of haematemesis
- Polyp (juvenile colonic polyp)
- Anal fissure
- Thrombocytopenia
- Colitis (e.g. ulcerative colitis, allergic colitis)

- Henöch–Schönlein purpura (HSP)
- Drugs
- Meckel's diverticulum
- Peptic ulcer
- Sexual abuse causing, for example, proctitis
- Swallowed blood (e.g. from epistaxis)
- Oesophagitis
- Haemolytic-uraemic syndrome (HUS)
- Inflammatory bowel disease

- Oesophagitis
- Lymphnodular hyperplasia

- Mallory–Weiss syndrome
- Familial adenomatous polyposis coli
- Haemangioma (50% have skin angiomas)
- Hereditary haemorrhagic telangiectasia
- Peutz–Jeghers syndrome
- Rectal foreign body
- Haemorrhoids

Differential diagnosis at a glance

	Any cause of haematemesis	Polyp	Anal fissure	Thrombocytopenia	Colitis
Diarrhoea	No	No	No	No	Yes
Massive bleed	No	Possible	No	Possible	No
Painless bleed	Yes	Yes	No	Yes	No
Vomiting	Yes	No	No	No	No
Bright-red blood	No	Yes	Yes	Possible	Yes

Recommended investigations

***   FBC: anaemia suggests chronic blood loss or acute massive bleeding or HUS. Anaemia with high CRP suggests inflammatory bowel disease. Low platelets is diagnostic in thrombocytopenia and disseminated intravascular coagulation.

***   Blood grouping if bleeding is massive.

***   LFTs may suggest liver cirrhosis. RFT showing high urea and creatinine suggests HUS.

***   Clotting study to evaluate coagulopathies such as haemophilia.

***   Apt test to differentiate maternal blood from fetal blood.

***   Stool testing for occult blood to confirm or exclude bleeding; culture will rule out infective colitis.

**   Abdominal plain X-ray is useful in suspected cases of necrotising enterocolitis or intussusception.

***   Sigmoidoscopy/colonoscopy indicated in suspected polyp: tumour or proctitis.

**   Air-contrast barium enema and nuclear scintigraphic imaging if the diagnosis remains unclear.

TOP TIPS

- Rectal bleeding in a healthy neonate is most often maternal blood in origin, swallowed during either delivery or breastfeeding.
- Neonatal peptic ulcer may be caused by hyperalimentation or drugs such as indomethacin

used for patent ductus arteriosus closure. Neonatal stress ulcer has often been linked with antenatal dexamethasone given for lung maturity in preterm infants.

- In paediatrics, anorectal disorders such as fissures, distal polyps and haemorrhoids are the most common causes of GI bleeding producing bright-red blood.
- Remember that juvenile colonic polyp (inflammatory polyp) is the most common GI tumour in childhood, affecting 3%–4%. The most common age at presentation is 2–8 years.
- GI bleeding is less common with Crohn's disease than with ulcerative colitis. The former presents with the triad of anaemia, loss of weight and abdominal pain.
- The two possible sources of rectal bleeding are an upper GI bleed (usually causing melaena) and a lower GI bleed (causing bright-red bleeding). However, massive upper GI bleeding can produce bright-red blood per rectum if the GI transient time is rapid.
- Important factors in the differential diagnosis of GI bleeding: age of the child, the presence or absence of anal pain during blood passage and the presence or absence of diarrhoea.
- Remember that not all red or black stools contain blood; iron, charcoal, liquorice, blueberries and bismuth preparations can cause a black appearance of a stool.

Red flags

- Beware of evidence of child sexual abuse presenting as GI bleeding, e.g. perianal trauma, tags or irregular or dilated anal tone and contour. Proctitis can also be caused by such forms of abuse.
- Although juvenile colonic polyposis is usually benign, dominantly inherited familial polyposis (familial adenomatous polyposis coli, Gardner's syndrome and Peutz–Jeghers syndrome) are pre-malignant polyps requiring resection (e.g. by snare cautery). Children with positive family history need supervision and genetic counselling.
- The abdominal pain in HSP may be severe and can lead to laparotomy, particularly if it precedes the skin rash and joint manifestations. Buttocks, arms and legs should be searched for urticarial lesions or petechiae.

NOTES:

DIARRHOEA

The clinician overview

Diarrhoea is very common in children and is most often infectious in origin. It is defined as an increase in the daily fluid losses of stool, which is usually associated with frequent stools. Most diarrhoeal diseases in children living in developed countries are viral, mild and self-limited, and do not require hospitalisation or laboratory evaluation. In developing countries, diarrhoea is often severe with a high death rate. In a young child who is ill enough to require hospitalisation, laboratory investigation of the stool is indicated to determine the cause of the diarrhoea.

Possible diagnoses

INFANTS
Common
- Physiologic in breastfed
- Milk protein/lactose intolerance
- Antibiotic induced
- Malabsorption (e.g. coeliac disease, cystic fibrosis
- Acute infective enteritis

Rare
- Botulism
- Primary disaccharide deficiency
- Acrodermatitis enteropathica
- Short bowel syndrome
- Munchausen's syndrome by proxy

CHILDREN
- Acute infective enteritis (viral and bacterial)
- Antibiotic-induced (e.g. pseudomembranous colitis)
- Postinfectious secondary lactose/protein intolerance
- Toddler's diarrhoea
- Malabsorption (e.g. coeliac disease, cystic fibrosis)

- Inflammatory bowel disease
- Overflow in constipation
- Irritable bowel syndrome
- Acrodermatitis enteropathica
- Munchausen's syndrome by proxy

Differential diagnosis at a glance

	Acute infective enteritis	Antibiotic-induced	Postinfectious secondary lactose/ protein intolerance	Toddler's diarrhoea	Malabsorption
Fever	Possible	No	No	No	No
Watery	Possible	Possible	Possible	No	Possible
Blood, mucous	Possible	Possible	Possible	No	No
Acute presentation	Yes	Yes	Possible	No	Possible
Thriving	Possible	Possible	Possible	Yes	No

Recommended investigation

** Blood U&E is indicated unless the diarrhoea is mild and there are no signs of dehydration.

*** Stool for culture (bacterial), and antigen for viral cause (rotavirus).

*** Testing the stool with a Clinitest tablet (to detect reducing substances such as lactose or glucose). Stool pH: in lactose intolerance it is acidic (pH < 5.5).

TOP TIPS

- The principal complication from diarrhoea is dehydration. If a child is alert and playful, the degree of dehydration is insignificant.
- Mothers are usually good historians. Simply asking about urine frequency and colour can give an important estimate of the degree of dehydration: concentrated urine (orange colour) suggests mild dehydration; an infrequent and small amount of urine suggests moderate dehydration. Anuria means severe dehydration.
- Diarrhoea persisting for more than 2 weeks (termed protracted or chronic diarrhoea) is mostly due to milk lactose or protein intolerance. Temporary withdrawal of milk and dairy products is usually diagnostic and therapeutic.
- Large watery diarrhoea in association with central abdominal pain and vomiting is typical of enteritis (usually termed gastroenteritis), whereas small, frequent stools and lower abdominal pain with blood in stool are very suggestive of colitis.
- Toddler's diarrhoea is common and may be misdiagnosed as gastroenteritis. These children are healthy and thriving, passing 3–5 soft stools daily, often containing undigested food particles (e.g. carrots, whole peas).
- In protracted diarrhoea, milk protein, lactose intolerance and Crohn's disease need to be excluded. Clinitest tablet is the simplest test to confirm or exclude lactose intolerance.

■ Children presenting with loose, frequent stools may have an infection elsewhere, e.g. urinary tract infection or appendicitis.

■ Laxative-induced diarrhoea (induced illness or Munchausen's syndrome by proxy) is rare but should not be missed. The diarrhoea is usually chronic or recurrent. There is an underlying psychiatric disturbance in the carer of the child.

NOTES:

CONSTIPATION

The clinician overview

Constipation is a common complaint that accounts for some 25% of visits to paediatric gastroenterologists. It is either functional (in 95% of cases) or organic (in 5% of cases). The latter often presents in the first few weeks of life. Constipation is a term used to describe infrequent defecation (fewer than three times per week) and a hard stool that is difficult to pass. It is important to remember that infrequent defecation is common in breastfed babies who may not have a stool for 10 days or even longer. There should be no intervention as long as babies are thriving, feeding well, have no abdominal distension and pass stools without pain or blood. Straining during defecation is normal. In older children, the most common reason is withholding stool for fear of having a bowel movement following an experience of painful defecation.

Possible diagnoses

INFANTS
Common
- Normal variant in breastfed
- Insufficient fluid intake, dehydration
- Neurodisability (cerebral palsy (CP), myotonica dystrophica)
- Intestinal obstruction (e.g. meconium ileus, plug)
- Hirschsprung's disease (HD)

Rare
- Persistent vomiting (e.g. pyloric stenosis)
- Metabolic (e.g. hypercalcaemia)
- Change from breastfeeding to bottle-feeding
- Intestinal stricture
- Anteriorly displaced anus
- Hypothyroidism
- Imperforate anus
- Any cause of polyuria (renal tubular acidosis)

CHILDREN
- Chronic habitual constipation
- Prolonged febrile illness
- Increased output (e.g. polyuria, vomiting)
- Neurodisability (CP, myotonica dystrophica)
- Irritable bowel syndrome (alternate with diarrhoea)

- Metabolic (e.g. hypercalcaemia, hypokalaemia)
- Recurrent or chronic vomiting
- Hypothyroidism
- HD
- Drugs, such as narcotics, antidepressants
- Lead poisoning
- Botulism

- Tethering of the spinal cord
- Other causes of muscular hypotonicity (botulism)

Differential diagnosis at a glance

	Chronic habitual constipation	Prolonged febrile illness	Increased output	Neurodisability	Irritable bowel syndrome
The only symptom	Possible	No	No	No	No
Associated dehydration	No	Possible	Possible	Possible	No
Mild constipation	Possible	Yes	Possible	Possible	Yes
History of loose stools	Possible	Possible	No	Possible	Yes
Short history	No	Possible	Possible	No	No

Recommended investigations

***   Urinalysis to exclude associated UTI.

***   TFT, serum calcium, U&E to exclude hypothyroidism, hypercalcaemia or hypokalaemia.

***   Serum lead level.

*   Plain abdominal X-ray that may show distended rectum (megacolon) full of faeces.

***   MRI for spinal cord disorders such as tethered spinal cord.

***   Rectal biopsy if there is clinical suspicion of HD.

TOP TIPS

- By far the most common cause of constipation is functional; organic diseases (HD, hypothyroidism, hypercalcaemia, renal tubular acidosis) are rare in practice.
- Looking at the child can give important clues to the underlying diagnosis, e.g. hypothyroidism, failure to thrive with distended abdomen in HD or Elfin face in hypercalcaemia.
- Parents usually wrongly interpret withholding stool as pushing. Doctors should give an explanation why this is not the case.
- Physical examination of a child with constipation should routinely include palpation of the abdomen for faecal mass, and anal and sacral areas for fissure and sacral anatomical abnormalities.
- Faecal soiling may be mistaken for diarrhoea. Parents should be given information about the mechanisms of soiling.
- Faecal soiling (involuntary seepage of a small amount of stool) is usually caused by chronic rectal retention and is treated by evacuating the rectum.

☑ Parents of constipated children should be told that long-term treatment is often required: while 60%–70% of children recover within 1–2 years, some 30% may expect a longer time with laxatives.

Red flags

☑ Over 90% of healthy neonates pass a stool in the first 24–48 hours of life, but waiting more than 48 hours is abnormal.
☑ Rectal examination (RE) is indicated in suspected HD: an empty rectum with palpable stool masses in the abdomen and a gush of air and liquid stool upon withdrawal of the examining finger may suggest the diagnosis.
☑ RE should not be a routine procedure. If this becomes necessary, explain the procedure and the reason for it.
☑ Beware that the rectum is normally empty or nearly so; a rectum full of hard stool suggests chronic constipation.
☑ Routine radiography and anorectal manometry are not recommended for evaluation of children with constipation.

NOTES:

JAUNDICE

The clinician overview

Jaundice (apparent if the total bilirubin is more than 35 μmol/L) is very common during the neonatal period. Almost all neonates become jaundiced with indirect hyperbilirubinaemia in the first few days of life. Jaundice appearing after 3 or 4 days of life suggests an infection, e.g. urinary tract infection (UTI) or sepsis. Jaundice after the first week of life suggests breast milk jaundice, biliary atresia, infection or metabolic disorders, e.g. galactosaemia or hypothyroidism. After the neonatal period, viral hepatitis remains the most common cause of jaundice worldwide. Hepatitis A virus (HAV) used to be a common infectious disease, but its incidence has declined significantly in developed countries. The prevalence of hepatitis B virus (HBV), hepatitis C virus (HCV) and other hepatotropic viruses has increased worldwide, causing chronic liver disease and primary hepatocellular carcinoma. An estimated 300 000 new cases of HBV infection occur in the United States alone each year. Jaundice should be differentiated from xanthochromia (carotenaemia), caused by carotene deposits in the skin.

Possible diagnoses

INFANTS
Common
- Physiological
- Haemolytic (e.g. ABO incompatibility)
- Breast milk
- Polycythaemia
- Parenteral hyperalimentation

Rare
- Congenital spherocytosis
- Congenital hepatitis (e.g. cytomegalovirus)
- Biliary atresia
- Metabolic (e.g. galactosaemia)
- Hypothyroidism

CHILDREN

- Infectious hepatitis (e.g. HAV, HBV)
- Drug-induced (e.g. paracetamol overdose)
- Malaria
- Mononucleosis
- Haemolytic anaemia

- Gilbert's syndrome
- Autoimmune hepatitis
- Hepatic abscess
- Reye's syndrome
- Leptospirosis
- Wilson's disease
- Brucellosis
- Obstructive jaundice (e.g. by gallstones)
- Yellow fever

- ◪ Cystic fibrosis
- ◪ Typhoid fever
- ◪ Liver cirrhosis
- ◪ Crigler–Najjar syndrome

Differential diagnosis at a glance

	Infectious hepatitis	Drug-induced	Malaria	Mononucleosis	Haemolytic anaemia
Fever	Possible	Possible	Yes	Yes	Possible
Anaemia	No	Possible	Yes	No	Yes
Splenomegaly	Possible	No	Yes	Possible	Possible
Lymphadenopathy	Possible	No	No	Yes	No
Abdominal pain	Yes	Possible	Possible	Possible	Possible

Recommended investigations

*** Urine: Clinitest for reducing substances will suggest galactosaemia, and culture to confirm UTI.

*** FBC: Hb low in haemolysis; leukocytosis suggests infection; reticulocytosis suggests haemolysis.

*** LFTs: direct hyperbilirubinaemia indicates hepatocellular disease such as hepatitis; indirect hyperbilirubinaemia with otherwise normal LFTs is very suggestive of Gilbert's syndrome, a transaminase level, alkaline phosphatase (increased in bile obstruction), prothrombin time, partial thromboplastin time and albumin level). Positive direct Coombs's test on the infant supports ABO and Rh incompatibility. Serological tests for hepatitis viruses.

*** Blood group and Rh status of the mother and infant.

*** Tests for intrauterine infections (TORCH).

*** TFTs to assess thyroid function.

*** Abdominal ultrasound scan to rule out bile obstruction (e.g. choledochal cyst) or mass.

** Other tests include isotope scan with technetium, percutaneous needle liver biopsy.

TOP TIPS

- ◪ Physiological jaundice occurs in most neonates during the first few days of life, it is not a disease; it is not present in the first 24 hours and it is always an indirect hyperbilirubinaemia.
- ◪ Breast milk jaundice is nothing other than physiological jaundice, which may persist for weeks. It is not a disease and mothers should be encouraged to continue breastfeeding.

- An infant with yellow skin but normal white sclera usually has carotenaemia, not jaundice.
- There is no evidence that a well full-term baby without haemolysis will get any ill effect from a bilirubin < 400 μmol/L.
- Direct-reacting bilirubin is water soluble, not fat soluble, and therefore it does not damage the brain tissue to cause kernicterus. It is, however, associated with serious diseases, such as congenital hepatitis and biliary atresia. The indirect bilirubin is fat soluble and may enter the brain tissue causing kernicterus.
- Gilbert's syndrome is the most common cause of indirect bilirubin jaundice in older children. It is a benign condition and should be differentiated from haemolytic anaemia (the latter has low Hb and high reticulocyte count).
- Although infectious hepatitis is the most common cause of jaundice worldwide, jaundice occurs in fewer than one in ten children with HAV, one in four with HBV and in less than one in three with HCV.
- Beware the extrahepatic presentation of a child with HBV infection: arthralgia, urticaria, arteritis, glomerulonephritis and aplastic anaemia.

Red flags

- There is a lack of correlation between bilirubin levels and kernicterus in preterm infants, i.e. kernicterus can occur at lower levels of bilirubin in these infants because of altered permeability of the blood–brain barrier by hypoxia, hypoglycaemia and other risk factors.
- A direct bilirubin of 34 μmol/L or greater indicates serious disease and is never physiological, e.g. neonatal hepatitis secondary to congenital infection (e.g. rubella, cytomegalovirus) or biliary atresia.
- It is urgent to determine the cause of direct hyperbilirubinaemia in an infant before irreversible damage to the liver occurs. The Kasai operation is most successful (rate of success is > 90%) if performed before 8 weeks of life.
- A neonate born to a HBsAg-positive mother should receive three HBV vaccines; the first one accompanied by 0.5 mL of hepatitis B immune globulin before leaving the baby nursery.
- A child with jaundice should not be diagnosed with hepatitis on the basis of hyperbilirubinaemia. An increased transaminase level is essential in diagnosing icteric and anicteric cases of hepatitis.

NOTES:

Bones and joints

Painful arm

Painful leg and limping

Arthralgia (painful joint)

Arthritis (swollen joints)

Myalgia (painful muscles)

PAINFUL ARM

The clinician overview

In children, arm pain usually results from musculoskeletal injuries (sprain, strain, contusion, dislocation and fracture). In the absence of dislocation and fracture, a musculoskeletal pain syndrome (MSPS) can be considered. The pain may affect part of the arm, the whole upper arm or the forearm, occurring suddenly or gradually, constantly or intermittently, and often associated with a burning or numbing sensation. If there is a history suggestive of injury (e.g. sport activity) the diagnosis is evident. A moderate to severe injury is likely to be followed by an inflammatory response that manifests as pain, spasm, reduced arm movement and redness and swelling. Less common causes of arm pain include neurovascular, cardiovascular disorders and referred pain from another area such as the neck, chest or abdomen.

Possible diagnoses

INFANTS
Common
- Birth injury
- Pulled elbow (nursemaid's elbow)
- Myalgia (e.g. viral infection)
- Child abuse
- Infection (osteomyelitis)

Rare
- Injury (dislocation, fracture)
- Bone tumour
- Scurvy
- Arthritis

CHILDREN
- MSPS
- Dislocation, fracture (including nursemaid's elbow)
- Myalgia (e.g. viral infection)
- Tendonitis and tenosynovitis
- Arthritis

- Injury (dislocation, fracture)
- Chronic fatigue syndrome (CFS)
- Fibromyalgia
- Reflex sympathetic dystrophy
- Cervical nerve root compression
- Malignancy (bone tumour)
- Osteomyelitis
- Neuritis (neuropathy)
- Raynaud's phenomenon (causes intermittent pain)

- Herpes zoster
- Scurvy
- Compartment syndrome
- Brachial plexus
- Spinal abscess

Differential diagnosis at a glance

	MSPS	Dislocation, fracture	Myalgia	Tendonitis and tenosynovitis	Arthritis
Non-arthritic pain	Yes	No	Yes	Possible	No
Usually mild pain	Yes	No	Yes	Possible	No
Associated swelling/ tenderness	No	Possible	No	Yes	Yes
Fever	No	No	Possible	No	Yes
Normal laboratory (e.g. WBC, CRP)	Yes	Yes	Possible	Yes	No

Recommended investigations

***   High FBC and CRP will support bacterial infection or arthritis.

**   Autoantibody screen is useful in case of Raynaud's phenomenon.

***   X-ray of the arm is very helpful in excluding fracture or dislocation.

***   Spinal X-ray is indicated if spinal lesions are suspected.

**   Bone scan in case of suspected osteomyelitis or malignancy.

TOP TIPS

- Muscle pain (myalgia) is common in association with many acute conditions such as viral infection, metabolic disorders, polyneuropathy and myositis.
- Pain in the elbow may be caused by nursemaid's elbow, caused by someone pulling hard on the child's hand or wrist.
- MSPS is a diagnosis of exclusion. Children have a normal physical examination except tenderness to light touch over several areas of the arm.
- Fibromyalgia and reflex sympathetic dystrophy are variant manifestations of MSPS. Although symptoms often overlap with MSPS they tend to be prolonged and recurrent.
- Although growing pain affects the lower extremities more often than the upper extremities,

arms may be involved. Remember its criteria: pain is episodic, typically nocturnal, non-articular, with no daytime disability, and continues for months.

- Compartment syndrome, though rare in children, affects circulation and function due to increased pressure in a confined space, causing severe pain to be felt with passive muscle stretching.
- In any child with a trauma, peripheral pulses and capillary refill time must be checked.
- When fatigue is a prominent feature and is more prominent than pain, consider CFS. Although children with MSPS may present with fatigue, this is likely to be mild.
- Children with fibromyalgia may present with symptoms of irritable bowel syndrome (incidence around 50%), migraine or tension headaches (incidence around 50%) or temporomandibular joint dysfunction.

Red flags

- The presence of paraesthesiae, such as numbness, suggests a neurological condition, e.g. neuritis, or nerve trapping. Beware that children may interpret paraesthesiae and muscle weakness as pain. Careful history taking and physical examination are essential.
- The possibility of child abuse, Munchausen's syndrome by proxy and school phobia should always be considered in the differential diagnosis for a young child who presents with unexplained pain.
- Beware that Raynaud's phenomenon can present with swelling and pain of the fingers and forearm. If this phenomenon worsens over time and is associated with skin changes, autoimmune diseases such as dermatomyositis, systemic scleroderma, or systemic lupus erythematosus could be the underlying cause.

NOTES:

PAINFUL LEG AND LIMPING

The clinician overview

Pain in the leg is common and caused by musculoskeletal disorders predominately as a result of trauma, developmental, infectious, rheumatological and neoplastical disorders. Painful limping is the usual presentation. These disorders may affect the hip (e.g. transient synovitis, avascular necrosis or slipped capital femoral epiphysis (SCFE)), knee (e.g. avascular necrosis, osteochondritis dissecans, and idiopathic adolescent knee pain syndrome), foot (e.g. poor-fitting shoes, trauma and avascular necrosis) and non-articular pain such as growing pain. The key to an accurate diagnosis is a careful history, thorough physical and neurological examination, and appropriate radiological and laboratory investigations.

Possible diagnoses

INFANTS
Common
- Birth injury
- Fracture
- Child abuse
- Infection (e.g. osteomyelitis)
- Arthritis/arthralgia

Rare
- Osteochondritis in syphilis
- Congenital hip dislocation

CHILDREN

- Trauma (minor muscle strains/sprains/overuse)
- Growing pain
- Transient synovitis
- Avascular necrosis (e.g. Perthes' disease)
- Arthralgia/arthritis (*see* Arthritis (swollen joints) section)

- Drugs (steroids)
- *Borrelia* (Lyme disease)
- Cerebral palsy (hemiplegia)
- Malignancy (leukaemia, lymphoma)
- Psychiatric diseases (e.g. conversion disorder)
- Sickle-cell anaemia
- Deep-vein thrombosis
- Gout
- Sciatica
- Dermatomyositis
- Polyneuropathy

Differential diagnosis at a glance

	Trauma	Growing pain	Transient synovitis	Avascular necrosis	Arthritis/ arthralgia
Musculoskeletal tenderness	Yes	No	Possible	Yes	Yes
Fever	No	No	Possible	No	Possible
Limping	Possible	No	Yes	Yes	Yes
Nocturnal pain	Possible	Yes	No	No	No
Diagnostic by X-ray	No	No	No	Yes	No

Recommended investigations

***   FBC and CRP are occasionally necessary: in infectious diseases (e.g. osteomyelitis, arthritis).

**   Rheumatoid factor, ANAs, human leukocyte antigen B27 are needed for rheumatological cases.

**   CPK, serum transaminases for muscular diseases.

***   TFTs and growth hormone level in pre-pubertal children with SCFE.

***   X-ray of the leg can diagnose many disorders, e.g. tumour or avascular necrosis.

**   MRI is sometimes needed as indicated by the result of the X-ray.

TOP TIPS

- The history of growing pain is diagnostic: non-articular pain occurring at night for at least 6 months and normal physical examination.
- Although individual avascular necrosis is uncommon, all together are common, particularly those affecting the hip (Perthes' disease) and the knee (Osgood–Schlatter disease).
- In a child with preceding upper respiratory tract infection who is afebrile with sudden limping, transient synovitis is very likely. Laboratory and radiological investigations are usually normal.
- Although X-rays of the leg are often requested for suspected cases of avascular necrosis (osteochondrosis), a more important reason is to exclude other lesions such as tumour.
- Don't forget that long-term use of steroids can cause osteoporosis, fractures and avascular necrosis.
- Before diagnosing a disease in a child with leg pain, examine for poor-fitting shoes or any foreign body such as a nail. These are common causes.
- Remember that imaging of the bone is normal in the early stages of Perthes' disease; the 'crescent sign' in a frog lateral position is the earliest possible radiological sign.
- Many children with hip diseases present with knee pain. Examination of all joints is essential.

▱ When the knee is examined, patellofemoral crepitations may be elicited. This is common in normal individuals and does not indicate a knee disease.
▱ SCFE is the most common hip disorder in adolescence; when it occurs pre-pubertally, an endocrine cause such as hypothyroidism or growth hormone deficiency may be the underlying pathology.

Red flags

▱ Any child with leg pain and limping needs proper evaluation to rule out serious causes such as tumour. An X-ray or other imaging technique is usually required.
▱ Perthes' disease is not uncommon in children; the prognosis depends on the age at clinical onset: those older than 10 years will almost certainly develop degenerative arthritis later on in life.
▱ In a young child with an unexplained pain, child abuse should not be forgotten in the differential diagnosis. Examine the skin carefully for relevant bruises; skeletal survey may be required.

NOTES:

ARTHRALGIA (PAINFUL JOINT)

The clinician overview

Arthralgia indicates joint pain not accompanied by obvious clinical signs of arthritis. It may be generalised involving multiple joints caused mostly by a viral infection, or involving the hip, knee, ankle or temporomandibular joint. The best approach to a child with arthralgia and normal examination is to perform careful initial evaluation and inflammatory tests (such as WBC, CRP) followed by periodic monitoring for changing symptoms or physical findings. Parents are usually worried that a rapid diagnosis often cannot be made and that clinicians are not telling them what is wrong with their child. Parental concern should be alleviated by informing the parents that there is a programme in place to monitor their child's symptoms.

(Arthralgia affecting the arms is discussed earlier in this chapter, *see* Painful arm section.)

Possible diagnoses

INFANTS
Common
- Acute viral infection
- Trauma
- Sickle-cell anaemia (SCA)
- Child abuse
- Malignancy (e.g. leukaemia, bone tumour)

Rare

CHILDREN
- Acute viral infection
- Trauma
- Hip pain (e.g. transient synovitis, Perthes' disease)
- Knee pain (e.g. chondromalacia, subluxation, osteochondritis)
- Ankle pain (e.g. sport injury, sprains)

- Pre-arthritis stage
- Malignancy (e.g. leukaemia, bone tumour)
- SCA
- Henöch–Schönlein purpura
- Child abuse
- Inflammatory bowel disease (Crohn's disease, ulcerative colitis)
- Rheumatic fever
- Sarcoidosis
- Drugs (e.g. carbimazole)
- Psychogenic

- Trichinosis
- Hypermobility of connective tissue
- Immunodeficiency (e.g. IgA deficiency)
- Wegener's granulomatosis

Differential diagnosis at a glance

	Acute viral infection	Trauma	Hip pain (e.g. transient synovitis)	Knee pain (e.g. chondromalacia patella)	Ankle pain (e.g. avascular necrosis)
Mono-arthralgia	No	Possible	Yes	Yes	Yes
Fever	Possible	No	Possible	No	No
Associated with or follows URTI	Yes	No	Yes	No	No
Usually adolescent age	No	possible	No	Yes	Possible
Diagnosed by an X-ray	No	Possible	No	No	Yes

Recommended investigations

***   FBC with CRP: elevated in bacterial diseases; leukopenia in systemic lupus erythematosus.

**   CPK: elevated in dermatomyositis.

***   Hb-electrophoresis and peripheral film for sickle-cell anaemia.

**   Kveim test for suspected cases of sarcoidosis.

***   X-ray: diagnostic for avascular necrosis and excludes other pathologies such as tumour.

**   Bone scan is sometimes required, e.g. suspected bone tumour.

TOP TIPS

- Arthralgia in association with acute viral illness should be considered as part of myalgia affecting the tissue surrounding the joints.
- Every attempt should be made to localise the arthralgia. Once a joint is found responsible, differential diagnosis becomes easy.
- Arthralgia of the hip includes transient synovitis (typically at age 3–7 years, child wakens with severe groin pain causing limping or refusal to walk), Perthes' disease or slipped capital femoral epiphysis. The latter affects typically obese, short children or those with a rapid growth spurt.
- Painful knee may be caused by traumatic synovitis, haemarthrosis, chondromalacia patella (also termed idiopathic adolescent anterior knee pain syndrome), patellar subluxation or dislocation, synovial plicae, osteochondritis dissecans or tumour.
- Patellar subluxation is not uncommon, detected when the knee is in full extension. Displacing the patella laterally results in the patient grabbing the examiner's hand (apprehension sign).
- Painful ankle may be due to sport injury (most common cause), referred pain from avascular necrosis of the navicular bone (Köhler's disease) or the metatarsal head (Freiberg's disease).
- Although persistent arthralgia without evidence of arthritis is uncommon in juvenile rheumatoid arthritis (JRA), arthralgia lasting several weeks may occur in the pre-arthritic stage of the disease.
- Although children with avascular necrosis of the tibia (Osgood–Schlatter disease) usually present with pain around the anterior knee, examination often reveals swelling, tenderness and prominence of the tibia tubercle. Healing is usually slow, taking 12–24 months.
- Remember that the diagnosis of JRA should only be made if there is evidence of arthritis (not arthralgia), persistent for more than 6 weeks and other diagnoses have been excluded.

- Before diagnosing arthralgia, ensure that there are no signs of arthritis (red, hot and swollen joint) and there is no obvious clinical evidence of effusion in the joint.
- Never forget that knee pain may be a referred pain originating from a diseased hip, such as transient synovitis. The detection of effusion in the knee is indicative of intra-articular process.
- The finding of haemarthrosis (usually in the knee) is indicative of a serious injury to ligaments, meniscus or occult fracture. Urgent referral to orthopaedic surgery is indicated.

NOTES:

ARTHRITIS (SWOLLEN JOINTS)

The clinician overview

A detailed discussion on arthritis, which comprises more than 100 different diseases, is beyond the scope of this book. In short, arthritis may be monoarthritis, oligoarthritis (< 5 joints) or polyarthritis (> 4 joints). The main causes of oligoarthritis are trauma, septic arthritis, juvenile rheumatoid arthritis (JRA), reactive arthritis (ReA), Lyme disease, transient synovitis, neoplastic and TB arthritis. Causes of polyarthritis include JRA, rheumatic fever (RF) and vasculitis. JRA and ReA are forms of autoimmune arthritis; the latter develops in response to an infection, occurring 1–3 weeks elsewhere in the body, and most commonly a viral upper respiratory tract infection (URTI) or intestinal infection (campylobacter, salmonella, or yersinia). JRA is classified into systemic-onset (associated with high remittent fever, rash, generalised lymphadenopathy, hepatosplenomegaly, serositis), oligoarthritis and polyarthritis.

Possible diagnoses

INFANTS
Common
- Postinfectious arthritis
- Septic arthritis
- Collagen disease
- JRA
- Vasculitis

Rare

CHILDREN

- Postinfectious arthritis (reactive, transient synovitis)
- JRA
- Collagen disease (e.g. systemic lupus erythematosus (SLE), dermatomyositis)
- Vasculitis (Henöch–Schönlein purpura, Kawasaki's disease)
- Septic arthritis (SA)

- Familial Mediterranean fever
- Trauma
- RF
- Arthritis of inflammatory bowel disease
- Lyme disease
- Neoplastic arthritis (leukaemia, lymphoma)
- TB arthritis

- Psoriatic arthritis
- Behçet's disease
- Reiter's syndrome

Differential diagnosis at a glance

	Postinfectious	JRA	Collagen disease	Vasculitis	SA
High fever > 39.0°C	Possible	Possible	Possible	Possible	Yes
Monoarthritis	Possible	Possible	Possible	No	Yes
Persistent for weeks	No	Yes	Possible	No	No
Associated skin rash	Possible	Possible	Possible	Yes	No
High ANAs	Possible	Possible	Possible	No	No

Recommended investigations

***   FBC: ESR, WBC, platelets raised in many rheumatic diseases, including JRA.

***   Autoantibodies, such as ANAs, positive in many rheumatic diseases.

***   IgM-RF negative usually negative in systemic onset disease.

***   Imaging X-ray, CT/MRI.

***   Bone scan: positive in early stage of SA and osteomyelitis and when routine X-rays are normal.

**   Bone marrow aspiration is diagnostic in suspected cases of neoplastic arthritis.

TOP TIPS

- When a child presents with arthritis, the first question should be: is it monoarthritis, oligoarthritis or polyarthritis? That alone can restrict the differential diagnosis.
- Transient synovitis is common and diagnosed by mild or absent fever, history of a viral URTI and one hip being affected. Child appears well, limping but still walking. WBC, CRP and ESR are usually normal; WBC count in the joint fluid is < 50 000 cells/mm (aspiration rarely necessary). It is self-limiting, usually lasting 1–3 weeks.
- SA is almost always monoarthritis. It is defined as positive joint fluid culture for bacteria and/or WBC count in the joint fluid of > 50 000 cells/mm (predominately polymorphonuclear cells) with or without positive blood culture (positive in about 50%).
- RF is characterised by migratory arthritis, occurring 2–3 weeks following an untreated group A beta-haemolytic streptococcal pharyngitis. Diagnosis is established by Jones criteria.
- Anti-nuclear antibodies (ANAs) are specific for nuclear constitutes. These are among the most important arthritis tests: they are positive in nearly 100% in mixed connective tissue disease, over 95% in SLE and about 50% in JRA.
- SA is characterised by an abrupt onset of fever and joint pain; fever is usually high

(> 39.5°C), with severe pain, restricted range of joint movement and refusal to walk.

- Systemic onset JRA can be diagnosed by the intermittent fever (ranging from 39.5°C to 41.2°C), often hectic, with a daily rise in the evening, then falling to normal in the morning. As the fever continues, the pattern may become double quotidian. Fever is usually associated with the occurrence of rash, generalised lymphadenopathy and splenomegaly.
- The most common non-infectious cause of pyrexia of unknown origin is JRA. The pattern of fever may be diagnostic: intermittent, often hectic, with a daily rise in the evening and then falling to normal in the morning.

Red flags

- In rheumatology, an early diagnosis of the type of arthritis may not be possible for weeks and months. For example, a diagnosis of ReA may change to JRA. Children who even fulfil the diagnostic criteria of JRA may develop, months or years later, classical symptoms and signs of irritable bowel disease with diarrhoea, anaemia and weight loss. Therefore, repeated evaluation is important.
- Children with oligoarthritic JRA and positive ANAs are at high risk of developing iridocyclitis; referral to an ophthalmologist is essential.
- Neoplastic arthritis, though uncommon, should always be borne in mind. Diagnostic clues include the presence of lymphadenopathy, hepatosplenomegaly, anaemia, thrombocytopenia, blast cells on the peripheral blood smear, pyrexia is usually mild (< 39.0°C) or absent. Bone marrow aspiration is diagnostic.
- In TB arthritis there is typically a lack of response to treatment with antibiotics, non-steroidal anti-inflammatory drugs or intraocular steroids. Diagnosis is by positive Mantoux test, with possible TB lesions in a chest X-ray and synovial biopsy.

NOTES:

MYALGIA (PAINFUL MUSCLES)

The clinician overview

Acute muscle pain (myalgia) is a very common complaint in association with many infections – mainly viral infections such as influenza types A and B, coxsakievirus A2 and A9. It is not due to systemic or local spread of the microorganisms, but rather due to interleukin-1 effect, which induces protein breakdown (proteolysis). Amino acids released during proteolysis can be metabolised within the muscle as a direct source of energy and are re-used for the synthesis of new proteins. Myalgia can also be due to musculoskeletal injury (sprains, strains, overuse, contusions), musculoskeletal pain syndrome (MSPS), myopathic (e.g. dermatomyositis) and neuropathic (Guillain–Barré syndrome).

Possible diagnoses

INFANTS
Common
- Birth injury (muscle pulling, fracture)
- Any febrile illness
- Child abuse
- Familial Mediterranean fever (FMF)
- Connective tissue disease

Rare
- Scurvy

CHILDREN
- Any febrile illness
- MSPS
- FMF
- Connective tissue disease (CTD)
- Chronic fatigue syndrome (CFS)

- Child abuse
- Fibromyalgia
- Lyme disease
- Acute polyneuropathy (Guillain–Barré syndrome)
- Metabolic disease
- CFS
- Dermatomyositis
- Drugs (statins, carbimazole)
- Porphyria
- Bornholm's disease
- Trichinosis
- Polymyalgia rheumatica

☑ Electrolyte imbalance
☑ Rhabdomyolysis
☑ Wegener's granulomatosis

Differential diagnosis at a glance

	Any febrile illness	MSPS	FMF	CTD	CFS
Diffuse	Yes	No	Yes	Possible	Yes
Fever	Yes	No	Yes	Possible	Possible
Presence of fatigue	Possible	Possible	Possible	Possible	Yes
Mainly infants and toddlers	Yes	Possible	No	Possible	No
Abnormal WBC and CRP	Possible	No	Possible	Yes	No

Recommended investigations

***   Urine: proteinuria SLE and FMF (proteinuria is the first sign of amyloidosis). Urine for porphyrins to confirm porphyria and rhabdomyolysis.

***   FBC may be helpful in showing leukopenia, thrombocytopenia and anaemia in SLE. Eosinophilia in helminthic infection such as trichinosis.

***   CRP (or ESR) is helpful for bacterial infections, CTD, dermatomyositis and FMF.

**   Autoantibodies such as ANA are helpful in CTD.

***   For trichinosis, serological studies (bentonite flocculation test) and muscle biopsy (showing larvae) will confirm the diagnosis.

***   Ultrasound scan and/or MRI is helpful in some inflammatory conditions such as dermatomyositis.

TOP TIPS

☑ Not all muscle diseases produce pain. Muscle diseases not associated with myalgia include muscular dystrophy and spinal muscular atrophies.

☑ Diagnostic criteria for FMF are recurring episodes of fever, pain in the abdomen (peritonitis), the chest (pleuritis) or the joints (arthritis) and muscles (myalgia).

☑ Clinicians should be aware that there are overlapping symptoms among MSPS, fibromyalgia, CFS and reflex sympathetic dystrophy.

☑ Fibromyalgia is associated with widespread pain and stiffness in the muscles, sleep disturbance, school absence and fatigue. The condition may need to be differentiated from CFS.

- Careful history-taking and examination is required to differentiate myalgia from arthralgia and muscle weakness.
- Although trichinosis is uncommon in children in this country, it is common worldwide. Children present with localised myalgia and fever. The clue is ingestion of raw or undercooked pork meat. Eosinophilia is present in the blood.

Red flags

- In any child with unexplained muscle pain, child abuse should be considered among the differential diagnosis. Skeletal survey may be needed to confirm it.
- A child with acute muscular weakness affecting the limb girdle muscles should be suspected of having dermatomyositis until proven otherwise. A peri-orbital rash is an important clue.
- Myalgia can be the presenting symptom of some serious diseases including bone tumour.

NOTES:

Cerebral

Headache

Sleep disorder

Tremor

Acute confusional state

Seizure

Neuromuscular weakness

Impaired consciousness (fainting, coma)

HEADACHE

The clinician overview

This is a very common problem, occurring in about 50% of children aged 7 years and 80% of children aged 15 years. It may be acute, acute recurrent, chronic recurrent or progressive, caused by minor viral infection or severe underlying disease such as central nervous system (CNS) infection or increased intracranial pressure (ICP). Therefore, careful evaluation of a child with headaches is essential. Infants or toddlers may present with irritability, unwillingness to play, crying while holding the head or vomiting. The most common cause of headache is an acute viral infection, migraine and tension headache. Migraine without aura is the most common type, defined as a headache lasting 1–72 hours, plus two of the following: bilateral or unilateral, pulsating, aggravated by routine physical activities plus at least one of the following: nausea and/or vomiting, photophobia or phonophobia. Tension headache is diagnosed with these criteria: headache lasting from 30 minutes to 7 days, in addition to two of the following: pressing/tightening, non-pulsating, mild-moderate intensity, bilateral location with no nausea or vomiting.

Possible diagnoses

INFANTS
Common

- Birth trauma causing cerebral irritability
- Viral infection
- Migraine
- Head injury
- Subdural haematoma (e.g. child abuse)

Rare

- CNS infection
- Increased ICP

CHILDREN

- Common viral infections
- Migraine
- Tension headache
- Head injury
- Sinusitis

- Eye strain
- CNS infection (meningitis, brain abscess)
- Brain haemorrhage (e.g. subdural haematoma)
- Increased ICP
- Mitochondrial disease such as MELAS
- Medications
- Seizure

- ◪ Hypertension
- ◪ Benign increased ICP (pseudotumour cerebri)

Differential diagnosis at a glance

	Common viral infection	Migraine	Tension headache	Head injury	Sinusitis
Fever	Possible	No	No	No	Possible
+ family history	No	Yes	Possible	No	No
Worse with routine activity	No	Yes	No	Possible	Possible
Both sides of head	Yes	Possible	Yes	Possible	Possible
Nausea/vomiting	Possible	Yes	No	Possible	Possible

Recommended investigations

The vast majority of children presenting with headaches do not require any investigation. The indication to use neuroimaging is discussed in this section.

TOP TIPS

- ◪ Remember that chronic headaches are rarely due to a significant disease.
- ◪ In families with a history of migraine, migraine variants are common and include cyclic vomiting, paroxysmal vertigo, restless legs, paroxysmal torticollis and abdominal migraine.
- ◪ Neuroimaging is not indicated on a routine basis in children with recurrent headaches and normal physical examination. It should, however, be considered with abnormal neurological examination, progressive headaches or coexisting seizure.
- ◪ Although analgesics such as paracetamol, ibuprofen and sumatriptan are effective first line of treatment in migraine, evidence-based treatment or prophylaxis is lacking.
- ◪ Although indication to use migraine prophylaxis includes missing more than 3 days of school in a month and/or 1–2 attacks per week, the quality of evidence available for such prophylaxis is poor (Cochrane Review 2010).
- ◪ It is simple to differentiate the two most common causes of headaches: migraine disrupts the child's activity; tension headache does not.

Red flags

- Benign ICP (pseudotumour cerebri) is characterised by increased ICP (e.g. headaches, vomiting and papilloedema) with normal CSF and ventricular size. Focal neurological signs are absent. Urgent referral for imaging and treatment is required.
- Although most causes of headaches in children are benign, it is essential to consider an underlying systemic disease: worsening headache presenting in the morning and increases by stooping or straining suggests increased ICP.
- Beware a history of excessive use of analgesic in individuals with migraine: the headache may be analgesic-induced or it can be rebound headache.
- An infant with cerebral haematoma often suggests abuse. Children may present with irritability, vomiting, bulging fontanel and focal seizure. Fundoscopy may show retinal haemorrhage. Neuroimaging is urgent.
- Remember that MELAS (mitochondrial encephalopathy, lactic acidosis and stroke-like episodes) may present with recurrent migraine headaches.
- Basilar migraine (presenting with vertigo, diplopia, blurred vision ataxia) should be differentiated from posterior fossa tumour.
- Alternating hemiplegia may be the first sign of later migraine. Beware that frequent vasoconstriction causing the hemiplegia causes ischaemia, which may lead to cerebral injury and developmental delay later on.

NOTES:

SLEEP DISORDER

The clinician overview

Children require sufficient sleep, although the amount required varies. Sleep duration mainly depends on age. Young infants need on average 14 hours of sleep per 24 hours, which is almost evenly distributed throughout the day and night. Children aged 6–12 years require about 10–11 hours and teens about 9 hours. It is fairly normal for infants to wake several times at night; some 30% of infants do this. Older children (4–12 years) commonly present with bedtime resistance. Insufficient sleep at night is likely to affect the child's mood and behaviour during the day, leading to school problems such as reduced attention span, aggressiveness and poor performance. Parasomnia is disruptive sleep-related disorders occurring during the NREM (non-rapid eye movement) sleep such as sleepwalking, sleep terrors and confusional arousal. Those disorders occurring during REM (rapid eye movement) sleep include absent sleep paralysis. Hypersomnia, or excessive sleep, includes narcolepsy.

Possible diagnoses

INFANTS
Common
- Any illness, any pain or discomfort
- Obstructive sleep apnoea syndrome (OSAS)
- Drugs
- Normal sleep patterns
- Improper sleep routines

Rare
- Pierre Robin sequence
- Congenital hypoventilation syndrome (Ondine's curse)

CHILDREN
- Insomnia for any illness, pain or itching
- Insomnia for improper sleep routines
- Anxiety
- Parasomnia (e.g. nightmares)
- Hypersomnia (e.g. narcolepsy)

- OSAS
- Side effects of drugs (methylphenidate), caffeine
- Kleine–Levin syndrome (KLS)
- Sleeping sickness (African trypanosomiasis)
- Periodic limb movement disorder (PLMD)
- Idiopathic hypersomnia

Differential diagnosis at a glance

	Insomnia for any illness, pain or itching	Insomnia for inadequate sleep routines	Anxiety	Parasomnia	Hypersomnia
Likely older child or adolescence	Possible	Possible	Yes	No	Yes
History is diagnostic	Yes	Possible	Possible	Yes	Yes
At night only	Possible	Yes	Yes	Yes	No
Attacks at REM sleep	No	No	Possible	No	Yes
Associated sleep paralysis	No	No	No	No	Yes

Recommended investigations

In the vast majority of cases, investigations are unlikely to be required.

** Polysomnography with oxygen saturation monitoring is very useful for insomnia evaluation, such as OSAS, narcolepsy and nocturnal seizures.

TOP TIPS

- Although many parents and clinicians often turn to medication to treat child insomnia, it is far more important to search for any underlying cause (e.g. anxiety) that needs to be treated first.
- Nightmares are differentiated from night terrors by easy recalling of the event in nightmares.
- Parents of children with night terrors are often woken by a piercing scream; the child looks flushed, frightened and agitated, and is not easily aroused. The child cannot recall the event the next morning.
- OSAS, which manifests as snoring and frequent cessation of sleep, is an important cause of insomnia. Children with Down syndrome, triangular chin and long soft palate are at risk of having OSAS. The child may need tonsillectomy and/or adenoidectomy.
- During sleepwalking, parents should not try to waken or restrain the child. Telling the child next morning about the event is unnecessary. If episodes are frequent, scheduled waking may help: the child is gently and briefly woken 15–30 minutes before the episode is due, and this is repeated for a month.
- Narcolepsy is characterised by recurring daytime sleepiness, often associated with disrupted sleep at night, cataplexy (loss of muscle control when, for example, laughing), sleep paralysis and hypnagogic phenomenon (auditory or visual illusion or hallucination when falling asleep).
- In contrast to narcolepsy, Kleine–Levin syndrome is rare. It is characterised by long and recurrent hypersomnia, hyperphagia and sometimes hypersexuality.

- Small infants have apnoea episodes at night; they are harmless and normal, lasting usually under 10 seconds and not associated with cyanosis, decreased oxygen saturation or bradycardia.
- Children with narcolepsy may not only present with daytime sleepiness but also with behaviour problems, irritability and deterioration of school performance.
- Narcolepsy is a lifelong problem. Although the tricyclic antidepressant clomipramine remains the main treatment, remember that it may cause numerous and unpleasant side effects: constipation, urinary retention and dry mouth.

Red flags

- Beware several sleep-related epileptic seizures: benign partial epilepsy with centrotemporal spikes (rolanic), benign epilepsy with affective symptoms, benign occipital epilepsy, and Panayiotopoulos syndrome. Autonomic symptoms and secondary generalisation may occur in these sleep-related epilepsies.
- Beware nocturnal frontal lobe epilepsy (NFLE), which may mimic night terrors. A child with NFLE has a variety of motor features (kicking, hitting, thrashing, cycling and scissoring of the legs) and vocalisation (shouting, grunting, screaming and coughing). EEG may help in establishing diagnosis.
- Sleepwalking occurs occasionally in 20%–40% and frequently in 3%–4% of the population; typical age is 4–8 years. Serious accidents may occur; securing the home (e.g. secured windows, locked doors) is essential.
- Excessive daytime sleepiness may be a sign of the existence of a major sleep disorder such as OSAS, idiopathic hypersomnia, PLMD, nocturnal seizures, KLS and narcolepsy.

NOTES:

TREMOR

The clinician overview

Tremor is a rhythmic, involuntary oscillation of part of the body, usually the hands, neck or head (titubation). It is classified as rest tremor (e.g. in Parkinson's disease or drug induced) and action tremor (occurring, for example, in cerebellar lesions). Rest tremor is noted when the hands are resting on the lap. Action tremor is produced by voluntary muscle contraction and is either postural (when affected arms are extended in front of the body) or target-directed movement such as intention. Tremor can be a manifestation of a serious neurological or metabolic disease. Tremor needs to be differentiated from ticks and chorea.

Possible diagnoses

INFANTS
Common
- Normal jitteriness
- Infants of maternal addiction
- Seizure (e.g. hypoglycaemia)
- Cerebral palsy
- Cerebral irritation

Rare

CHILDREN

- Physiological tremor
- Essential tremor (autosomal dominant)
- Anxiety
- Medications (e.g. β-2 agonists for asthma)
- Cerebellar disease

- Cerebral palsy
- Acute confusional state (*see* Acute confusional state section)
- Writing tremor
- Hyperthyroidism
- Wilson's disease
- Juvenile Parkinson's disease
- Spinocerebellar ataxia
- Acute intermittent porphyria

Differential diagnosis at a glance

	Physiological tremor	Essential tremor	Anxiety	Medications	Cerebellar disease
+ family history	Possible	Yes	Possible	No	Possible
Postural	Yes	Yes	Yes	Possible	No
Normal examination otherwise	Yes	Yes	Yes	Possible	No
Progressive	No	Possible	No	No	Possible
Diagnosis by history	Possible	Possible	Possible	Yes	Possible

Recommended investigations

***   Urine for copper and serum ceruloplasmin for cases with Wilson's disease.
***   Urine for toxicology from a neonate, and if possible from the mother.
***   TFT for suspected hyperthyroidism.
***   Imaging of the brain for cerebral or cerebellar causes.

TOP TIPS

◩ Jitteriness, a rhythmic tremor of equal amplitude, is very common in healthy neonates, particularly premature infants and crying babies.

◩ In a child with tremor, examination should be performed while the child is at rest, with arms outstretched and while reaching for targets.

◩ Physiological tremor probably occurs in most individuals when the arms are extended. This is enhanced by anxiety, stress or caffeine. More subtle tremor can be demonstrated by holding a piece of paper in outstretched hands.

◩ Drugs causing tremor include amphetamine, asthma medications such as β-2 agonist and theophylline, and anticonvulsants such as valproate and tricyclic antidepressants.

◩ Beware that essential tremor may be unilateral.

◩ The bronchodilator β-2 agonist salbutamol is by far the most common drug causing tremor and tachycardia. Although these are benign, parents should be made aware of them at the time the drug is prescribed to avoid parental anxiety.

◩ Tremor needs to be differentiated from tics, which are actually jerks, non-rhythmic and can affect any muscle. Chorea is usually symmetric, more rapid than tremor, jerky and predominately affects the face.

Red flags

- Drug addiction (e.g. cocaine, heroin, amphetamine) among pregnant women has increased steadily over years. The result is increased incidence of neonatal withdrawal syndrome with irritability, jitteriness and occasionally seizures. Obtaining a detailed maternal drug history is essential.
- Jitteriness in neonates needs to be differentiated from seizure caused by, for example, hypoglycaemia or hypocalcaemia. Normal jitteriness has no abnormal gaze or eye movement, bradycardia or tachycardia; it is provoked by stretching a joint and stops on holding of the limb.
- Beware that jitteriness may be a manifestation of prenatal exposure to maternal marijuana or neonatal withdrawal effect from other illicit narcotic use. Taking detailed maternal history is essential. Babies of women who smoke more than five marijuana cigarettes weekly during gestation demonstrate marked tremors and startles, which are attenuated by 30 days.
- In any child with progressive or acute tremor, serious conditions such as Wilson's disease, hyperthyroidism, hypoglycaemia, hypocalcaemia, neuroblastoma and phaeochromocytoma have to be excluded.

NOTES:

ACUTE CONFUSIONAL STATE

The clinician overview

Acute confusional state (ACS) is characterised by sudden alteration of the mental state leading to an inappropriate interaction with people and environment. A child presenting with ACS should be regarded as a medical emergency. It is characterised by an acute and dramatic onset of disorientation, impaired concentration and subtle motor signs such as tremor. Disorientation of time is most common in older children. In the absence of a relevant medical history (such as sickle-cell anaemia or medication), the differential diagnosis can be quite difficult and challenging for clinicians to make. ACS should be differentiated from delirium. In delirium, there is extreme disturbance of arousal, attention, orientation and perception, most commonly accompanied by fear and agitation. Delirium is often associated with fever.

(In infants, ACS occurs as an alteration of consciousness and is discussed later in this section.)

Possible diagnoses

INFANTS
Common

CHILDREN

- ☑ Migraine
- ☑ Side effect of medication
  (e.g. antihistamine, antiepileptic drugs
  (AEDs))
- ☑ Encephalitis/encephalopathy
- ☑ Non-convulsive status epilepticus
  (NCSE)
- ☑ Psychosis

Rare

- ☑ Head injury
- ☑ Hypoglycaemia
- ☑ Brain tumour
- ☑ Night terror
- ☑ Systemic lupus erythematosus (SLE)
- ☑ Brain haemorrhage
- ☑ Metabolic disorder
- ☑ HIV infection

- Malignant hypertension
- Cerebral venous sinus thrombosis
- Carbon monoxide poisoning

Differential diagnosis at a glance

	Migraine	Side effect of medication	Encephalitis/ encephalopathy	NCSE	Psychosis
Previous or associated headaches	Yes	Possible	Possible	No	Possible
+ family history	Possible	No	No	Possible	Possible
Fever	No	Possible	Possible	Possible	No
Terminate after sleep	Yes	Possible	No	Possible	No
Abnormal EEG record	Yes	No	Yes	Yes	No

Recommended investigations

***   Blood glucose to exclude hypoglycaemia.

***   Serological tests to exclude SLE.

***   EEG for seizure (such as NCSE) or encephalitis.

***   Neuroimaging with MRI or CT scan for head injury, encephalitis (such as herpetic encephalitis).

TOP TIPS

- Treatment of ACS is directed at the underlying systemic problem including withdrawal of any offending toxin and drugs, and correcting metabolic errors as soon as possible.
- EEG is diagnostic in NCSE: administration of IV AEDs will normalise the EEG and recover ACS.
- The first step in evaluating any child with psychosis: are they on any medication? In adolescence, illicit drugs (cocaine, amphetamine and ecstasy) are a common cause.
- A confusional state of migraine often lasts several minutes to hours. It may be the first presentation before being replaced by typical migraine attacks.
- The diagnosis of the first episode of acute confusional migraine is often difficult; drug abuse, encephalitis and NCSE need to be considered. Family history of migraine, severe headaches or visual symptoms prior to the confusion may suggest the diagnosis.
- Psychosis has many underlying causes. The role of clinicians is to exclude a medical problem such as psychosis that should be urgently referred to psychiatric services.
- Remember that haloperidol is often used to treat ACS. The drug can cause unpleasant extra-pyramidal side effects. Procyclidine is an effective antidote.

Red flags

▱ Psychosis has numerous neurological causes including brain tumour, central nervous system infection and, most important in adolescents, drugs such as amphetamine, cocaine and ecstasy. Mental psychosis should include symptoms such as delusion, hallucination and paranoid ideation.

▱ Be aware that minor trauma can occasionally trigger a major ACS grossly disproportionate to the degree of trauma.

▱ NCSE should be considered in all children with ACS whether or not there is a history of epilepsy.

▱ Remember that psychiatric manifestations in patients with SLE (personality changes, depression and psychosis) are prominent. Laboratory testing for SLE is urgently required.

NOTES:

SEIZURE

The clinician overview

Seizures are common in the paediatric population, occurring in 5%–7% of children. The normal organised tonic-clonic seizure patterns seen in older infants and children are not seen in neonates. Seizure patterns in neonates include focal clonic, multi-focal jerks, apnoea eye blinking and jitteriness. In older children, febrile seizures (FS) are the most common cause of seizures occurring in 3%–4%, followed by epileptic seizure. Epilepsy should not be diagnosed unless seizures recur and they are unprovoked (e.g. by fever). The term 'seizure' is used in preference to 'convulsion' as some seizures have no abnormal convulsive movements. Any seizure has to be differentiated from pseudoseizure occurring with conversion symptoms.

Possible diagnoses

INFANTS
Common
- Hypoxic-ischaemic encephalopathy (HIE)
- Cerebral haemorrhage
- Metabolic (e.g. hypoglycaemia, hypocalcaemia)
- Infection (e.g. meningitis)
- Developmental/malformation

Rare
- Fifth-day seizure (benign idiopathic neonatal seizure)
- Inborn errors of metabolism
- Mitochondrial disease
- Menkes' kinky hair disease

CHILDREN
- FS
- Epilepsy (generalised and partial)
- Metabolic
- Infection
- Pseudoseizure

- Cerebral haemorrhage
- Intracranial tumours
- Drug induced

Differential diagnosis at a glance

	Febrile seizure	Epilepsy	Metabolic	Infection	Pseudoseizure
Fever	Yes	No	No	Yes	No
Duration commonly < 5 minutes	Yes	Possible	Possible	Possible	Possible
+ family history	Possible	Possible	No	No	No
Previous episode	Possible	Yes	Possible	No	Possible
Usually generalised	Yes	Possible	Yes	Possible	Possible

Recommended investigations

*** Blood: FBC, CRP, blood culture, electrolytes, glucose, calcium, magnesium, urea.

*** Prolactin blood level if pseudoseizure is suspected (high in genuine seizure).

*** EEG for afebrile seizures.

*** Neuroimaging for cases in whom an intracranial lesion is suspected (encephalitis, abscess, focal seizures, complex partial seizures, and increased intracranial pressure).

TOP TIPS

- ☑ Seizures occur during the neonatal period more than at any other period in children because of the high incidence of infections, trauma to the brain, structural lesions of the brain and metabolic disorders. HIE is the most common cause of neonatal seizures.
- ☑ Evaluation of a child with seizure should focus upon a search for an organic and treatable cause.
- ☑ The first step in an evaluation is to determine whether it is seizure or conditions that mimic seizures. These conditions include breath-holding attacks, benign paroxysmal vertigo, syncope, narcolepsy and pseudoseizures.
- ☑ FS is a benign condition provoked by a sudden rise of fever. Investigation in an otherwise healthy child is unnecessary except for urine examination. The minimum work-up for the first unprovoked seizure in an otherwise healthy child is blood tests for glucose, calcium, magnesium, electrolytes and urea, and an EEG.
- ☑ Neuroimaging may not be necessary in primary generalised epilepsy, simple febrile seizure, Rolandic type and typical absence seizures.
- ☑ Seizures occurring during the initial phase of sleep or on waking in an older child are suggestive of benign partial epilepsy with cenro-temporal (Rolandic) spikes (10%–15% of all childhood epilepsy) or juvenile myoclonic epilepsy (5%–10% of all childhood epilepsy).
- ☑ Counselling the parents and children with seizures should include purpose and side effects of the medications (to improve compliance) and first-aid measures in case the seizure recurs.
- ☑ EEG is a frequently abused and misinterpreted investigation. It is an aid to the clinical diagnosis and classification of epilepsy. Typical absence seizures that can be reproduced

by hyperventilation do not necessarily need this investigation. EEG, on the other hand, is essential for any child with focal seizures.

- Pseudoseizure can sometimes be difficult to differentiate from epileptic seizure: video recording and serum prolactin (increased in true epilepsy) can help.

Red flags

- In neonatal seizures, subsequent developmental delay, cerebral palsy, epilepsy and death are related to low Apgar scores at 5 minutes (particularly the presence of hypotonia), prolonged seizure, unresponsiveness to antiepileptic drugs (AEDs) and the need for more than one AED to control the seizure.
- FS should be differentiated from meningitis; children with central nervous system infection are usually unwell with lethargy, headache, anorexia and vomiting before the onset of the seizure.
- Hypomagnesaemia (magnesium < 1.5 mg/dL) is very often associated with hypocalcaemia. The seizure will not respond to calcium treatment but an injection of intramuscular magnesium will correct both conditions.
- Any type of seizure may develop into status epilepticus (SE); generalised tonic-clonic is the most common cause. Omission of taking anticonvulsant drugs is another important cause of SE.

NOTES:

NEUROMUSCULAR WEAKNESS

The clinician overview

Weakness is a decreased ability to voluntarily and actively move muscles against resistance. It may arise from any portion of the motor unit, which consists of a neuron in the cortex and its corticospinal tract (both forming the upper motor neuron, UMN), anterior horn cell, peripheral nerve, neuromuscular junction and muscle (all forming the lower motor neuron, LMN). Cerebral palsy is excluded from neuromuscular disorders (NMD). A UMN lesion may manifest as intellect deficits, decreased muscle power (palsy and not paralysis), increased muscle tone (spasticity), hyperactive reflexes, myoclonus and intact sensation. An LMN lesion may manifest as normal intellect, markedly reduced muscle power (paralysis), reduced muscle tone and reflexes and fasciculation (present with anterior horn cell disease). Weakness must be differentiated from hypotonia, fatigue and ataxia.

Possible diagnoses

INFANTS
Common
- Cerebral and spinal cord injuries
- Hypoxic ischaemic encephalopathy
- Congenital myopathies (e.g. central core disease)
- Central nervous system infection and malformation
- Traumatic facial palsy

Rare
- Congenital muscular dystrophy
- Congenital myasthenia gravis
- Familial dysautonomia (Riley–Day syndrome)
- Alternating hemiplegia

CHILDREN
- Muscular dystrophies (Duchenne's, myotonic)
- Migraine hemiplegia
- Neuropathies (e.g. Guillain–Barré syndrome)
- Neuromuscular junction diseases (e.g. myasthenia)
- Todd's paralysis (following a seizure)

- Metabolic myopathies
- Cerebral or spinal tumour
- Botulism
- Poliomyelitis
- Hypothyroid and hyperthyroid myopathy
- Periodic paralysis (hyper- and hypokalaemic)

- Drugs (e.g. steroids)
- Motor neuron disease
- Transient myelitis

Differential diagnosis at a glance

	Muscular dystrophies	Migraine hemiplegia	Neuropathies	Neuromuscular junction diseases	Todd's paralysis
Proximal muscle weakness	Yes	No	No	No	No
History of seizure	No	No	No	No	Yes
Affecting the cranial nerves	No	No	Possible	Yes	No
Progressive weakness	Yes	No	Possible	Yes	No
Specific treatment available	No	Possible	Possible	Yes	Possible

Recommended investigations

*** Electrolytes for unexplained episodic paralysis.

*** TFT in suspected thyroid-related disorders.

*** Serum creatine phosphokinase for muscle diseases.

*** Anti-acetylcholine antibody in plasma and IV edrophonium will confirm myasthenia.

*** Neuroimaging for suspected cerebrovascular diseases.

*** EMG can differentiate between neuropathic and myopathic disorders.

** Muscle biopsy.

TOP TIPS

- Examination of a child with weakness should always begin with observation, including the head (shape and size), face (for dysmorphism), eyes (for strabismus, ophthalmoplegia), skin and muscles (for any lesion, atrophy, hypertrophy, fasciculation) and gait (waddling, ataxic) and difficulty in rising up from the floor.
- A frequent under- and postgraduate examination case is a child with hemiplegia. Diagnosis is easy by observing the gait with one arm held flexed and adducted against the chest while the leg is circumducted.
- Remember that proximal muscle weakness (shoulders and hips) indicates a myopathy, while distal weakness (hands) indicates a neuropathy. Myotonic dystrophy is an exception, with weakness affecting the hands.
- Both hypothyroidism and hyperthyroidism can cause proximal muscle myopathies; patients with Graves' disease may cause ophthalmoplegia.
- Hypotonia may be due to weakness or without weakness (e.g. Down syndrome). Weakness is excluded by a normal antigravity power, i.e. lifting a limb remains elevated.
- Remember that some children, such as those with leukodystrophies, usually have both UMN and LMN lesions, so localising a single lesion may not be possible.
- Because specific therapy is available for many NMDs and because of genetic and prognostic implications, accurate diagnosis with the help of investigation is essential.

- Hemiplegic migraine may be either sporadic or inherited as autosomal dominant. Repeated attacks can lead to ataxia due to cerebellar degeneration.
- Beware that walking is defined as an achievement of six steps. Inability to walk by the age of 18 months may indicate an NMD. Serum creatine phosphokinase to exclude muscular dystrophy should be checked.
- Children with periodic paralysis are normal between episodes. Later these become more frequent, causing permanent weakness.
- Minor head injury is one of the most common causes of hemiplegic migraine attack. Avoidance of contact sports is important.

NOTES:

IMPAIRED CONSCIOUSNESS (FAINTING, COMA)

The clinician overview

Impaired consciousness may be brief or prolonged, mild or profound. Brief unconsciousness occurs with vasovagal syncope (transient, self-limited loss or consciousness or awareness) seizures, breath-holding attacks, head injury and cardiac arrhythmia. The latter, such as long QT syndrome (QT interval > 460 milliseconds), is an important cause of loss of consciousness and may mimic epilepsy. Prolonged and deeper impaired consciousness (coma) usually results from severe intracranial (e.g. infection, haemorrhage) and metabolic (e.g. diabetic ketoacidosis) disorders.

Possible diagnoses

INFANTS
Common
- Infection
- Seizures
- Head injury
- Breath-holding spells
- Intracranial haemorrhage

Rare
- Toxins/poisoning/medication
- Cardiac arrhythmia

CHILDREN

- Vasovagal faint
- Seizure (febrile seizure, epilepsy)
- Head injury
- Infection
- Breath-holding spells (cyanotic and pallid)

- Toxins/poisoning/medication
- Diabetic ketoacidosis/hypoglycaemia
- Intracranial haemorrhage
- Hysteria
- Electrolytes disturbance (e.g. hyponatraemia)
- Cardiac arrhythmia
- Narcolepsy

Differential diagnosis at a glance

	Vasovagal faint	Seizure	Head injury	Infection	Breath-holding spells
Likely > 10 years of age	Yes	No	No	No	No
< 1 minute	Yes	Possible	Possible	No	Possible
Fever	No	Possible	No	Yes	No
Often cyanosis	No	Yes	Possible	Yes	Possible
Diagnosis by history	Possible	Possible	Possible	Possible	Yes

Recommended investigations

*** FBC and CRP: leukocytosis and high CRP in infection.

*** Lumar puncture and BC for central nervous system infection.

*** Blood sugar (using BM stick) to diagnose hyper- or hypoglycaemia.

*** Tilt-table testing: very useful in children with unexplained syncope.

*** ECG in fainting to exclude prolonged QT; 24-hour continuous ECG is often required.

*** Plain X-ray for skull injury, skeletal survey for suspected abuse.

*** EEG and neuroimaging for suspected epilepsy, haemorrhage or mass.

TOP TIPS

◪ Most causes of impaired consciousness can be diagnosed from the history alone; so an eyewitness account is essential, e.g. if the event occurred at school, a report from there is required.

◪ A brief impairment of consciousness is likely to be either syncope or seizure.

◪ Glasgow coma scale is a valuable tool in assessing children with an altered level of consciousness, particularly in cases with head trauma.

◪ Diagnosis of breath-holding spells is easy from the history: both types (cyanotic and pallid) are triggered by an upsetting or painful event; impaired consciousness is often followed by tonic seizure.

◪ Long QT syndrome is either autosomal dominant inherited (Romano–Ward syndrome), autosomal recessive (Jervell and Lange–Nielson syndrome) or acquired (myocarditis or electrolyte disturbance).

◪ Before diagnosing epilepsy, consider conditions that mimic seizures such as breath-holding spells, syncope, narcolepsy and pseudoseizure. Remember that the latter frequently occurs in patients with past history of epilepsy. EEG and serum prolactin (increased in true epilepsy) help.

- ☑ Beware of head injury in infants: the majority of serious intracranial injuries (excluding road traffic accident) during the first year of life are due to abuse.
- ☑ Vasovagal syncope may be associated with brief tonic contraction, abnormal movements, upward eye deviation and even urinary incontinence. These should not be mistaken for epilepsy.
- ☑ Arrhythmias are an important cause of loss of consciousness and possible death; urgent referral to a cardiologist is indicated for consideration of treatment with β blockers. In refractory cases an implantable pacemaker or cervicothoracic sympathectomy should then be considered.
- ☑ Some SIDS (sudden infant death syndrome) cases are caused by long QT syndrome; parents and siblings should undergo ECG examination to exclude the abnormality.

NOTES:

Chest

Respiratory noises

Acute shortness of breath (dyspnoea)

Cough

Coughing up blood (haemoptysis)

Chest pain

Palpitation

Breast enlargement in boys (gynaecomastia)

Breast lumps

Nipple discharge

RESPIRATORY NOISES

The clinician overview

Although respiratory noises as reported by the parents are extremely common, these noises are often difficult to differentiate from one another. The difficulty is compounded by the fact that children may have multiple noises, being intermittent and changing from one noise to another in a few minutes or according to awake or sleep positions (polyphonic). Clinicians dealing with children should realise that it is very common that when parents report a type of noise, e.g. wheezing, it is often not confirmed. It is important to know that snuffles and stridor are caused by obstruction of the extrathoracic airways (nose, pharynx, larynx and the extrathoracic portion of the trachea), while wheezing is caused by intrathoracic obstruction. Clinicians should be familiar with a few common noises (wheeze, stridor, rattle, grunt, snore and snuffle) and be able to diagnose them. An error in recognising specific noises will lead to diagnostic and therapeutic errors.

Possible diagnoses

INFANTS
Common
- ☑ Snuffles
- ☑ Stridor
- ☑ Grunt
- ☑ Wheeze
- ☑ Rattle

Rare
- ☑ Mew

CHILDREN

- ☑ Wheeze
- ☑ Stridor
- ☑ Grunt
- ☑ Rattle
- ☑ Snore

- ☑ Snuffle
- ☑ Purr
- ☑ Moan
- ☑ Squeak

Differential diagnosis at a glance

	Wheeze	Stridor	Grunt	Rattle	Snore
Ill-looking	Possible	Possible	Yes	No	No
Expiratory	Yes	No	Yes	Yes	No
Inspiratory	Possible	Yes	No	Yes	Yes
Associated cough	Yes	Possible	Possible	Possible	No
Worse during sleep	Yes	Yes	Yes	Possible	Yes

Recommended investigations

**   FBC: leukocytosis in bacterial disease; BC if the stridor is suspected to be caused by epiglottitis.

***   Blood for chromosomal analysis if cri-du-chat is suspected.

**   Chest X-ray often required with more persistent symptoms.

***   Lung function tests useful in wheezy children; peak flow measurement in those over 5 years of age.

***   Direct laryngoscopy for unusual features of stridor.

**   Video recording the respiratory noises by the parents to help establish a diagnosis.

TOP TIPS

◪ Acute snuffles are mostly caused by a viral infection, while persistent ones may be due to allergic rhinitis, adenoid hypertrophy or 'normal' snuffly noises of infancy.

◪ Note that extrathoracic obstruction produces inspiratory stridor while the intrathoracic obstruction produces wheeze.

◪ When parents report their child has a wheeze, the child may have rattles or stridor. This must be confirmed. Be prepared to imitate a wheeze, stridor or whoop or ask parents to imitate the sound.

◪ A rattle should not be considered an asthma symptom; if acute it is due to viral infection, if persistent it is due to GO reflux or sputum retention, often found in neuromuscular diseases.

◪ The association of hoarseness and stridor suggests an obstruction at the vocal cords of the larynx such as laryngotracheobronchitis. Hoarseness in laryngomalacia is not present because vocal cords are not involved. When cough is also present, the trachea is involved.

◪ Laryngomalacia is the most common cause of chronic stridor, noted usually soon after birth, and disappears at the age of 12–18 months. It is not associated with cough, failure to thrive or feeding problems. It does not need a laryngoscopy to confirm it unless there are atypical features.

◪ Cri-du-chat is a rare syndrome producing unusual sounds. This is due to a deletion of the short arm of chromosome 5 and is characterised by a high-pitched, mewing cry, resembling a kitten.

- Beware that persistent snuffles (inspiratory nasal) are so common in early infancy that they can be regarded as normal. They are often misdiagnosed as cold. Their disappearance is expected at around 4–6 months of age.
- Persistent nasal snuffles need to be differentiated from partial choanal atresia. In older children, polyps need to be excluded. In case of polyps, cystic fibrosis is high on the list as a cause.

Red
flags

- In contrast to other respiratory noises, expiratory grunt is usually a serious sign seen in neonates in association with respiratory distress syndrome and in older children with pneumonia.
- A major error is missing an upper airway obstruction and misdiagnosing stridor as a wheeze.
- A missed diagnosis of inhalation of a foreign body or of cystic fibrosis can have significant implications for the child, as these can cause bronchiectasis, abscess and severe pneumonia.
- The term 'snuffles' was first used for children with congenital syphilis. Although this infection is rare, it is on the rise and should not be missed. Typical presentation is the triad of anaemia, snuffle and splenomegaly.

NOTES:

ACUTE SHORTNESS OF BREATH (DYSPNOEA)

The clinician overview

Dyspnoea is a subjective feeling of difficulty in breathing. Children may describe dyspnoea as 'getting easily tired', or 'can't keep up with other kids'. It may occur spontaneously or during certain activities such as exercise or during feeding in infants. Dyspnoea is a common symptom of a variety of cardio-pulmonary diseases. Respiratory diseases, such as asthma, remain the most common reason for dyspnoea. Congestive cardiac failure (CCF) is the second-most-common cause of dyspnoea at any age of childhood. In older children, psychological factors can contribute to the sensation of dyspnoea. Children presenting with dyspnoea usually have other symptoms and signs of respiratory distress syndrome, including tachypnoea, subcostal recession and tachycardia. The term may also include 'unusual pattern of breathing'. For example, hyperpnoea, which occurs in metabolic acidosis, such as diabetic ketoacidosis, may also give a sensation of dyspnoea.

Possible diagnoses

INFANTS

Common

- Respiratory distress syndrome
- Transient tachypnoea
- Viral-induced wheeze
- Bronchiolitis
- Congestive cardiac failure

Rare

- Pulmonary oedema
- Pneumonia
- Pneumothorax
- Persistent pulmonary hypertension
- Pleural effusion
- Pulmonary hypoplasia
- Pericardial tamponade

CHILDREN

- Asthma
- Viral-induced wheeze/bronchiolitis
- Pneumonia
- CCF
- Psychogenic

- Pulmonary oedema
- Obstructive airway diseases
- Pulmonary embolism
- Inhaled foreign body
- Chronic lung disease
- Neuromuscular disease (e.g. myasthenia gravis)
- Hyperventilation
- Pulmonary embolism

Differential diagnosis at a glance

	Asthma	Viral-induced wheeze/ bronchiolitis	Pneumonia	CCF	Psychogenic
Grunting	No	No	Yes	No	No
Tachypnoea	Yes	Yes	Yes	Yes	No
Wheeze	Yes	Yes	No	Possible	No
Low O_2 saturation	Possible	Possible	Possible	Possible	No
Reduced peak flow	Yes	Possible	Possible	Possible	No

Recommended investigations

*** O_2 saturation, peak flow measurements and, in severe cases, blood gases.
*** Lung function tests to differentiate between obstructive (decrease in flow) and restrictive (decreased lung volume) causes of dyspnoea.
*** Chest X-ray: may show hyperinflation (asthma), collapse or consolidation or pneumothorax.
*** Echocardiography and ECG in patients with suspected heart disease.

TOP TIPS

◪ Dyspnoea rarely occurs in isolation. Accompanying features include cough, wheezing, tachypnoea and subcostal recession.

◪ A clear distinction between bronchiolitis and bronchitis in the first 2 years of life is difficult and of no therapeutic significance.

◪ The question whether or not to admit a child with dyspnoea can be difficult. As a guide, O_2 saturation in air of more than 95% and peak flow measurement of more than 70% of the expected amount suggest that the child can be managed with medications at home.

◪ Asthma can have some shadows in the chest X-ray; these do not indicate pneumonia and will disappear with anti-asthmatic treatment.

◪ When an adolescent presents with hyperventilation, ask about other psychosomatic complaints, e.g. any problem with swallowing. The patient, often a girl, may describe swallowing difficulty, so-called globus hystericus.

◪ The differentiation between cardiac and pulmonary causes of dyspnoea can be difficult. The presence of murmur, liver enlargement and relative tachycardia are in favour of cardiac causes.

◪ An aid to differentiate cardiac from pulmonary dyspnoea is the hyperbaric oxygen test of breathing 100% oxygen. In pulmonary diseases there will be a normalisation of the O_2 saturation.

◪ The most common cause of dyspnoea is asthma. An accurate technique of delivering the bronchodilator, by observing the child using the inhaler, is essential.

◪ The history of a child with shortness of breath is incomplete without asking about symptoms associated with activities such as running and bike riding or exposure to cooler weather.

◪ Dyspnoea during exercise is frequently caused by asthma. Measurement of the peak flow before and after the exercise can help establish the diagnosis.

Red flags

◪ An infant with no murmur detected at birth but found to have a murmur at the age of 6 weeks with respiratory distress is likely to have CCF due to large ventricular septal defect (VSD). Symptoms should not be misdiagnosed as bronchiolitis.
◪ Wheezing is not a symptom of pneumonia, while grunting with flaring of alae nasi is a very important sign of pneumonia.
◪ A cardiac cause of dyspnoea is likely in a neonate who becomes dyspnoeic during feeding.

NOTES:

COUGH

The clinician overview

Cough is one of the most common symptoms in children. It has been estimated that children living in developed countries attend medical services five times a year and approximately half of them do so because of cough. Cough as a symptom is ubiquitous for almost the entire respiratory system. It may be a symptom of extrapulmonary disease, such as myocarditis or congestive cardiac failure. For practical purposes, cough is defined as acute (< 2 weeks) and subacute or chronic (> 2 weeks). Cough has to be persistent daily to be defined as chronic. Chronic cough is subdivided into specific cough (in the presence of identifiable respiratory disease or known cause) and nonspecific cough (absence of respiratory disease or known cause). Cough is also divided into dry (e.g. asthma) and wet/moist (bronchiectasis). Prescribing medications to suppress the cough is not part of paediatric practice, but finding the underlying cause of cough is essential.

Possible diagnoses

INFANTS
Common
- ☑ Upper respiratory tract infection (URTI)
- ☑ Lower respiratory tract infection (LRTI)
- ☑ Viral-induced wheeze
- ☑ Aspiration
- ☑ GO reflux

Rare
- ☑ Tracheo-oesophageal fistula
- ☑ Bronchiectasis
- ☑ Congenital lobar emphysema
- ☑ Pertussis

CHILDREN
- ☑ URTI (e.g. viral URTI, croup)
- ☑ LRTI (e.g. pneumonia, bronchitis)
- ☑ Asthma
- ☑ Allergy (dust or pollen inhalation)
- ☑ Psychogenic

- ☑ Ciliary dyskinisia
- ☑ Inhaled foreign body (FB)
- ☑ Cystic fibrosis (CF)
- ☑ Drugs (angiotensin-converting enzyme inhibitor)
- ☑ Alpha-1 antitrypsin deficiency
- ☑ TB
- ☑ Oesophageal-tracheal fistula
- ☑ Severe chest wall deformity

Differential diagnosis at a glance

	URTI	LRTI	Asthma	Allergy	Psychogenic
Associated wheeze	No	Possible	Yes	Possible	No
The only symptom	No	No	No	Possible	Yes
Runny/blocked nose	Yes	No	Possible	Yes	No
Associated fever	Yes	Yes	Possible	No	No
Low O_2 saturation	No	Yes	Yes	Possible	No

Recommended investigations

**   FBC: raised WBC in bacterial infection and sometimes in viral LRTI and asthma. Eosinophilia in allergic conditions.

**   Sputum for culture from children with productive cough.

***   Lung function testing: peak flow measurement helps in the diagnosis: before and 15 minutes after inhaled bronchodilator: this should show an improvement of at least 20%.

***   Chest X-ray is very helpful in diagnosing pneumonia, foreign body. Also very useful in excluding pathology if the presentation does not suggest a clear diagnosis.

***   CT scan: to diagnose bronchiectasis.

***   Sweat test if CF is suspected.

**   Children with chronic unexplained cough may require more sophisticated investigations, including bronchoscopy, video fluorescence and echocardiography.

***   Gastric pH study for cases suspected of having GO reflux.

TOP TIPS

- If the cough is persistent and a diagnosis has not been established, a trial with a bronchodilator is worthwhile; sometimes an inhaled steroid is helpful.
- Children's cough is rarely productive, therefore the term 'wet cough' rather than 'productive cough' is more appropriate.
- Cough is almost always originating from the respiratory system; an URTI is the most common cause.
- Cough without wheeze in asthma is rare but may occur.
- In a child with pertussis-like cough who is fully immunised, adenovirus and other viruses may have caused the illness.
- A psychogenic cough is rare but may occur; remarkably it never occurs during sleep.
- All children with chronic cough should have lung function tests, chest X-ray and O_2 saturation performed.
- Beware that a child who presents with cough only on exertion could have a mild asthma or heart disease. Peak flow measurements before and after exercise and with and without salbutamol inhalation will help establish the diagnosis of asthma.

▱ Cough is usually self-limited and the focus should be directed at the cause rather than at the treatment. Educate parents that 'cough medicines' will unlikely help children with cough.

Red flags

▱ Remember that FB can mimic symptoms of URTI, croup and asthma. For any young child with prolonged unexplained cough, a diagnosis of an inhaled FB should be excluded. If missed, bronchiectasis is likely to ensue.
▱ An underweight child with chronic cough should undergo a sweat test to exclude CF.
▱ A severe coughing paroxysm causing high intrathoracic pressure and reduced venous return and manifesting as red face may result in cerebral hypoxia and syncope.
▱ Some children with asthma produce abundant secretions causing wet cough. This can resemble cough in patients with CF.
▱ Beware that children with developmental delay may present with persistent cough due to aspiration and aspiration pneumonia. The cough can mimic the cough of asthma or bronchitis.

NOTES:

COUGHING UP BLOOD (HAEMOPTYSIS)

The clinician overview

Haemoptysis is defined as coughing or expectoration of blood or the presence of blood-tinged sputum. It is always a frightening experience for patients and their parents. However, in contrast to adults, haemoptysis is not a common symptom in children and is usually not life-threatening. There are numerous causes of haemoptysis, which can usually be diagnosed by obtaining a careful history, physical examination and laboratory testing. Infection is the most common cause (60%–70% of cases) and acute lower respiratory tract infection (LRTI) is the leading cause of infection. In general, the source of the bleeding is either from the lungs or the bronchial system. The amount of bleeding from the lung tissue tends to be small compared with the bleeding from the bronchi, which produce a greater quantity of blood. Haemoptysis must be differentiated from epistaxis and haematemesis.

Possible diagnoses

INFANTS
Common
- Side effect of pulmonary surfactants
- Post-intubation
- Disseminated intravascular coagulation
- Coagulopathy
- Pulmonary oedema

Rare
- Pulmonary oedema
- Cardiac failure
- Pulmonary tumours (e.g. adenoma)

CHILDREN
- Pneumonia
- Coagulopathy
- Cystic fibrosis (CF)
- Vigorous cough
- Foreign body (FB) (mostly under 4 years of age)

- Blunt-force trauma secondary to lung contusion
- Bronchiectasis
- Pulmonary embolism (PE)
- Pulmonary oedema
- Lung abscess
- TB
- Left-ventricular heart failure (cardiac haemoptysis)
- Goodpasture syndrome

- Hydatid cyst
- Wenger's granulomatosis
- Hereditary haemorrhagic telangiectasia
- AV (arterio-venous) malformation
- Eisenmenger's syndrome
- Pulmonary tumours (adenoma, haemartoma)
- Sarcoidosis
- Connective tissue diseases (particularly systemic lupus erythematosus)
- Haemosiderosis
- Mycetoma (fungus ball)

Differential diagnosis at a glance

	Pneumonia	Coagulopathy	CF	Vigorous cough	FB
Massive bleeding	No	Possible	No	No	Possible
Short history	Yes	Possible	No	Yes	Yes
Associated fever	Yes	No	Possible	Possible	Possible
Bleeding elsewhere	No	Yes	No	No	No
Previous haemoptysis	No	Yes	Possible	No	No

Recommended investigations

*** FBC: low Hb confirms anaemia if the bleeding is massive; leukocytosis in infection such as pneumonia or autoimmune diseases; low platelets in thrombocytopenia or coagulopathy.

*** Coagulation study with INR, PT and PTT.

** pH: an alkaline suggests haemoptysis and an acid will suggest haematemesis.

** D-dimer: elevated in pulmonary embolism.

** Auto-antibody screen may be positive for connective tissue diseases.

** Sputum cytology for suspected TB or tumour.

*** Chest X-ray is the most valuable investigation for detecting the majority of causes.

*** Sweat test for suspected cases of CF.

** Bronchoscopy and high-resolution CT scan of the lung may be indicated in unclear cases of haemoptysis such as tumour.

TOP TIPS

- Haemoptysis in young children is usually caused by benign conditions such as vigorous cough.
- After a careful history and physical examination, a chest X-ray should be performed. If the diagnosis is not clear, bronchoscopy, chest CT scan and referral to a chest specialist should be considered.
- A child with haemoptysis and high fever most likely has pneumonia.
- The low-pressure pulmonary system tends to produce a non-profuse haemoptysis while the bronchi, which are at systemic pressure, tend to produce more massive bleeding.
- Haemoptysis (with history of lung disease, frothy, bright-red expectoration, absence of nausea and vomiting) should be easily differentiated from haematemesis (with history of gastric or hepatic disease, coffee-ground, brown to red expectoration, presence of nausea and vomiting, mixed with food particles).
- Haemoptysis occurs in 5% of all patients with CF and may recur.
- While fibroptic bronchoscopy is preferred if a neoplasm is suspected, rigid bronchoscopy is the preferred investigation for massive bleeding because of its greater suctioning and airway maintenance capability.
- Paediatricians may manage children with haemoptysis if the diagnosis is clear, e.g. pneumonia. Unclear cases should be referred to a chest unit to establish the diagnosis and treatment.

- In any child with haemoptysis, CF is a possible cause; finger clubbing is an important clue.
- Beware that young children under 5 years of age swallow their sputum without apparent haemoptysis, unless the haemoptysis is massive.
- Beware FB as a cause of haemoptysis; it is the second-most-common cause after infection.
- Beware that among obscure causes of haemoptysis is left-ventricular heart failure or mitral stenosis causing pulmonary hypertension.
- Pulmonary embolism may cause haemoptysis. Consider this diagnosis if there is evidence of deep-vein thrombosis or the risk of thrombosis, such as sickle-cell anaemia or homocystinuria.
- TB is on the increase in the United Kingdom; the disease should not be forgotten as a cause of haemoptysis.

NOTES:

CHEST PAIN

The clinician overview

Chest pain is a common complaint in children. It is the second-most-frequent cause of referral to paediatric cardiologists after cardiac murmur. Although chest pain in adults is considered a medical emergency because of possible associated heart attack, in children this is fortunately not the case. Common causes include idiopathic, injury, musculoskeletal myalgia, pulmonary diseases (e.g. asthma), psychogenic and gastrointestinal disorders. Many teenagers present with psychogenic chest pain reflecting anxiety generated by some events. Others teenagers have chest pain because of benign transient intercostals muscle spasm. Chest pain can be acute or chronic; the latter lasts by definition longer than 6 months. Although chronic or recurrent chest pain is likely to be benign (mostly caused by anxiety), this complaint often leads to numerous school absences, restriction of normal activities and considerable worry to patients and their parents.

Possible diagnoses

INFANTS
Common
- Inflammatory changes (cellulitis)
- Child abuse (e.g. rib fracture)
- Trauma/injury
- Pneumonia
- Chest drain (therapeutic)

Rare
- Acute chest syndrome (sickle-cell anaemia (SCA))
- Anomalous origin of the coronary arteries
- Kawasaki's disease
- Scurvy

CHILDREN

- Idiopathic
- Anxiety/stress
- Costochondritis
- Direct trauma to the chest
- Pulmonary (pneumonia, asthma, pleurisy)

- Acid reflux
- Myositis (such as dermatomyositis)
- Ischaemic heart disease (e.g. Kawasaki's disease)
- Marfan's syndrome (because of the dissecting aortic aneurysm)
- Cardiac (e.g. aortic stenosis, pericarditis after coxsakievirus infection)
- SCA (causing ischaemic chest pain)
- Bornholm disease
- Herpes zoster

Differential diagnosis at a glance

	Idiopathic	Anxiety/stress	Costochondritis	Direct trauma to the chest	Pulmonary
Abnormal chest findings	No	No	Yes	Possible	Yes
Previous episodes	Possible	Possible	No	No	No
Likely under 10 years of age	Possible	No	No	No	No
Antecedent viral URTI	No	No	Yes	No	Possible
Localised (non-diffuse)	Possible	Possible	Yes	Possible	Possible

Recommended investigations

Laboratory tests are generally not helpful in establishing a specific cause for chest pain. In a few cases, the following tests may be required.

**   FBC may show anaemia in SCA.

***   Chest X-ray for cases of pericarditis, pneumonia chest syndrome for SCA.

***   ECG and 24-hour ECG if cardiac cases.

***   Echocardiography (with two-dimensional and Doppler echocardiography) for cardiac diseases.

**   Endoscopy if a gastric source of the pain is suspected (GO reflux).

TOP TIPS

- The first clinical issue in a child with chest pain is to decide whether the history and clinical findings suggest an organic or non-organic cause.
- Although chest pain in infancy is difficult to diagnose, few diseases (e.g. acute chest syndrome in SCA, anomalous origin of the coronary arteries and Kawasaki's disease) present with sweating, restlessness and crying as equivalent signs for expressing chest pain.
- Idiopathic chest pain is the most common cause, reported to occur in 20%–45% of cases. This is defined by absence of cause after thorough history, physical examination and laboratory testing.
- Chronic or recurrent episodes of chest pain of longer than 6 months without abnormal findings are likely to be psychogenic. This cause accounts for 5%–10% of cases and more commonly in girls.
- Costochondritis (Tietze's syndrome), frequently caused by viral infection, is characterised by localised swelling of the costo-chondral, costo-sternal or sterno-clavicular joints, mostly involving the second and third ribs. Chest movements or deep breaths may worsen the pain.

- Acid or GO reflux can cause retrosternal or left-sided chest pain with or without epigastric pain, often presenting as a burning sensation.
- Typical symptoms for psychogenic cause of chest pain: dull or sharp, of short duration and unrelated to exercise. Teenagers are mostly affected. Inquire about loss of a relative, pending examinations, bullying at school, break-up of relationship with a friend or a parent or close relative having had angina or a heart attack.
- A complaint of chest pain, discomfort or heaviness is suggestive of exercise-induced bronchospasms. A bronchodilator, such as a salbutamol inhaler, before the exercise is likely to prevent these symptoms and suggest the diagnosis.

Red flags

- A diagnosis of idiopathic or anxiety-related chest pain should be made only after excluding organic disease. Cardiac or pulmonary disease can occasionally be the underlying cause.
- Cardiac diseases causing chest pain/discomfort, dizziness and syncope include severe aortic stenosis, atrial myxoma (associated with tuberous sclerosis), hypertrophic cardiomyopathy, long QT syndrome and supraventricular tachycardia with very rapid heart rate.
- When a child presents with chest pain, and the history reveals a familial trait for hypertrophic cardiomyopathy, this diagnosis and referral to a paediatric cardiologist should be considered.
- Patients with Marfanoid appearance and chest pain require close attention because of the risk of dilatation of the ascending aorta and dissecting aneurysm. Referral to a cardiologist is urgent.

NOTES:

PALPITATION

The clinician overview

Cardiologists may use the term of palpitation to describe an awareness of the heartbeat due to abnormality of the heart rhythm ranging from simple, benign ectopic atrial or ventricular beats to more important tachy-arrhythmias. Patients may use the term to describe a perception or awareness of irregular, fast or skipped heartbeats or simple awareness of their pulse, particularly when it is fast or when lying on one side in bed. In paediatric practice, the differential diagnosis is usually narrowed between tachycardia (such as supraventricular tachycardia (SVT)) and ectopic beats. Any palpitation with a history of syncope without warning is most likely of cardiac origin (ventricular tachycardia (VT)). In such cases, an urgent evaluation is essential. Palpitation may be a terrifying experience for a child and for their parents. A young child who cannot explain the event by words may stop their normal activity, expressing discomfort or clutching the left side of the chest.

Possible diagnoses

INFANTS
Common

CHILDREN

- ▨ Sinus tachycardia (fever, exercise)
- ▨ Anxiety
- ▨ Anaemia
- ▨ Arrhythmia (such as ectopic beats, SVT)
- ▨ Drugs (e.g. β-2 agonists, use of stimulants)

Rare

- ▨ Thyrotoxicosis
- ▨ Heart diseases, such as heart block, hypertrophic cardiomyopathy, mitral valve prolapse)
- ▨ Excessive coffee
- ▨ Electrolytes disturbance
- ▨ Phaeochromocytoma
- ▨ Carcinoid syndrome

Differential diagnosis at a glance

	Sinus tachycardia	Anxiety	Anaemia	Arrhythmia	Drugs
Short, few minute episode	Possible	Possible	No	Possible	No
Regular rhythm	Yes	Possible	Yes	No	Possible
Associated pallor	No	No	Yes	Possible	No
Diagnosis requires ECG	No	No	No	Yes	Possible
Associated tremor	No	Possible	No	No	Yes

Recommended investigations

***   FBC to check the Hb for anaemia.

***   TFTs to diagnose hyperthyroidism.

***   U&E: to check for potassium level as electrolyte abnormalities may aggravate arrhythmia.

***   A chest X-ray may be helpful showing cardiac enlargement in case of failure.

***   ECG may establish the diagnosis of arrhythmia, e.g. SVT, sinus tachycardia or WPW syndrome; 24-hour ECG (Holter monitor) if the child was asymptomatic at presentation.

**   Treadmill exercise test may help reveal any exercise-induced arrhythmia.

TOP TIPS

☑ If the history suggests arrhythmia and examination is normal, the parents can be requested to bring the child during an attack for an ECG to establish a diagnosis.

☑ Most patients with palpitation do not have a cardiac lesion.

☑ Parents may be taught how to measure the pulse rate; this may be useful in cases of SVT.

☑ In considering the differential diagnosis of palpitation, the focus is on tachycardia (most important, SVT) or ectopic beats.

☑ Ectopic beats are benign, provided there is no evidence of a heart disease, anaemia or thyrotoxicosis.

☑ Sudden onset of tachycardia in association with dizziness and dyspnoea is almost diagnostic of SVT.

☑ While VF (ventricular fibrillation) causes unconsciousness, VT may be tolerated and present with palpitation and syncope.

☑ Beware that the normal pulse of a young infant under 3 months of age while awake ranges between 100 and 220 per minute. Sinus arrhythmia is so universal that it is abnormal for a child not to have it.

☑ If an underlying cause for the palpitation is not found, have a low threshold to refer the child to a paediatric cardiologist.

☑ A child with palpitation who is pale with a heart murmur should not be diagnosed as having cardiac disease; the murmur is likely to be a haemic functional murmur, which disappears once the anaemia is corrected.

- Palpitation is more serious if it is associated with chest pain, shortness of breath, fainting or cardiac disease. Urgent evaluation in these cases is needed.
- Although seeing a patient during an attack of palpitation is usually diagnostic, between attacks, the heart and ECG may be entirely normal. An exception to this is WPW syndrome associated with SVT.
- Beware that an SVT in a young child may present with congestive cardiac failure (CCF). Even if the child has not developed CCF, he or she will do so unless the SVT is converted soon to sinus rhythm.

NOTES:

BREAST ENLARGEMENT IN BOYS (GYNAECOMASTIA)

The clinician overview

Gynaecomastia is defined as a benign diffuse enlargement of the breast due to presence of mammary tissue, mainly glandular proliferation, in the male. It is the result of oestrogen–androgen imbalance (lack of testosterone or increase in oestrogen). While oestrogen stimulates breast tissue growth, androgen inhibits it. Diagnosis of gynaecomastia is made from medical history and physical examination. This is a common condition affecting the majority of male children at puberty, which is usually mild and resolves spontaneously. This type of gynaecomastia needs to be differentiated from obesity-related breast enlargement (pseudo-gynaecomastia), which is composed of adipose tissue (and not glandular tissue), medicated-induced gynaecomastia, familial gynaecomastia and local lesions inside the breast such as tumour.

Possible diagnoses

INFANTS
Common
- ☑ Physiologic (maternal hormones)
- ☑ Mastitis
- ☑ Drugs

Rare

CHILDREN

- ☑ Puberty (about two-thirds of all boys)
- ☑ Drugs (exposure to oestrogen)
- ☑ Familial gynaecomastia (autosomal dominant)
- ☑ Klinefelter's syndrome
- ☑ Obesity

- ☑ Growth hormone therapy
- ☑ Neurofibromatosis
- ☑ CAH (11β-hydroxylase deficiency)
- ☑ Thyroid disease (hypo- or hyperthyroidism)
- ☑ Adrenal tumour (feminising tumour)
- ☑ Hypogonadism and cryptorchidism
- ☑ Testicular tumour (leydig cell tumour)
- ☑ Testicular failure

- Prolactinoma
- Liver tumours (fibrolamellar tumour)
- Liver cirrhosis
- Peutz–Jeghers syndrome
- McCune–Albright syndrome
- HIV infection
- Breast carcinoma
- Androgen insensitivity syndrome
- Reifenstein's syndrome

Differential diagnosis at a glance

	Puberty	Drugs	Familial gynaecomastia	Klinefelter's syndrome	Obesity
Learning difficulty	No	No	No	Yes	No
Hypogonadism	No	No	No	Yes	No
Unilateral	Yes	Possible	Possible	Possible	No
Noted at puberty	Yes	No	No	Yes	No
Spontaneous resolution	Yes	No	No	No	Possible

Recommended investigations

***   TFT to assess thyroid function.

***   Hormonal assay: testosterone, LH, FSH and eostradiol: high LH level and low testosterone indicates testicular failure; low LH and testosterone indicate increase in oestrogens; high LH and testosterone indicate androgen resistance or neoplasm-secreting gonadotrophins.

***   17-hydroxyprogesterone and other tests for CAH. Prolactin level for hyperprolactinaemia.

***   Karyotyping if Klinefelter's syndrome. This is confirmed by an extra X chromosome.

***   Imaging: ultrasound scan for breast, renal and testicular masses. MRI scan for more detailed adrenal and pituitary imaging. MRI for suspected cerebral lesions (e.g. prolactinoma).

**   Biopsy for suspected breast or testicular tumours.

TOP TIPS

- Beware that enlargement of the breasts occurs in most neonates, males and females, as a result of stimulation by maternal hormones. It requires no investigation. Often there is some discharge from the nipple (colostrums). The discharge should not be squeezed or pressed to avoid infection. Spontaneous regression in a few days is the rule. Parents need to be reassured.

- During puberty, about two-thirds of boys develop breast enlargement, which may be unilateral and tender; complete resolution is the rule.
- In obese boys the breasts are enlarged due to fat tissue accumulation (pseudo-gynaecomastia), which may mimic gynaecomastia. In gynaecomastia, a firm or rubbery disc of tissue can be felt; in adipose tissue no such disc of tissue is present.
- The mean hormonal concentrations of FSH, LH, prolactin, testosterone and eostradiol are in boys with gynaecomastia are the same as in boys without it.
- Surgical removal of the enlarged breast is rarely indicated except by marked enlargement that has caused emotional stress to the child.
- Drugs known to cause gynaecomastia include ketoconazole, digoxin, methyldopa, furosemide, marijuana, spironolactone, oestrogen and anti-androgen drugs.
- If a drug is suspected to cause gynaecomastia, it should be discontinued, if possible, and patients attend a review appointment in a month. If the gynaecomastia was drug-induced, some reduction of the breast and disappearance of the discomfort are expected.
- Beware that pubertal gynaecomastia may be tender, unilateral; both are transient and resolve completely in 12–18 months.
- In any child with gynaecomastia, every effort should be made to exclude exposure to oestrogen, accidental or therapeutical. Increased pigmentation of the nipple and areola is an important clue.
- Klinefelter's syndrome is common (1 per 500–1000 of newborn males, making it the most common chromosomal aberration), and is associated with gynaecomastia in 80% of cases. The risk of breast cancer is 16 times higher than in other men. Monitoring the gynaecomastia is important.

Red flags

- Gynaecomastia associated with neurological manifestations such as progressive headaches and visual disturbance could be caused by pituitary tumour. An MRI scan is urgently required.
- In any child with gynaecomastia, testicular examination is essential to exclude tumour or testicular failure.
- Beware that any gynaecomastia with galactorrhoea (spontaneous flow of milk) may suggest the presence of prolactinoma as the underlying pathology; obtain urgently a serum prolactin level and head MRI.
- Breast cancer is rare and accounts for less than 1% of cancers in men. It presents as unilateral, hard to firm mass that is fixed to underlying tissue.

NOTES:

BREAST LUMPS

The clinician overview

Breast development starts normally in girls aged 8.5–13.5 years in five stages and is completed in late teens and early 20s. The vast majority of breast masses in children are benign and self-limited. Neonatal bilateral breast hypertrophy due to maternal hormonal influence is a very common finding in both sexes. Breast buds and thelarche may occur in female toddlers; the condition is usually benign if it occurs in isolation. Nonetheless, a lump in the breast is an alarming sign because parents associate any breast swelling with cancer. A thorough history and physical examination, sometimes requiring needle aspiration and biopsy, are essential in any child who has a mass in the breast.

Possible diagnoses

INFANTS
Common
- Bilateral breast enlargement
- Mastitis/abscess
- Haemangioma
- Cyst
- Injury to the breast

Rare

CHILDREN
- Thelarche (including premature thelarche)
- Breast buds
- Precocious puberty
- Benign tumour (e.g. fibroadenoma, haemangioma)
- Breast engorgement

- Trauma
- Drugs (oestrogen, systemic or topical)
- Intramammary lymph node
- Malignant tumours (rhabdomyosarcoma, non-Hodgkin's lymphoma, metastatic neuroblastoma)
- Virginal hypertrophy (macromastia)
- Fibrocystic (mammary dysplasia)
- Lipoma
- Fat necrosis
- Macromastia

Differential diagnosis at a glance

	Thelarche	Breast buds	Precocious puberty	Benign tumour	Breast engorgement
Often unilateral	Yes	Yes	Possible	Yes	Possible
Adrenarche present	No	No	Yes	No	No
Growth spurt	No	Yes	Yes	Possible	Yes
Isolated round mass	No	Yes	No	Yes	Yes
May affect toddlers	Yes	Yes	Yes	Possible	No

Recommended investigations

*** Hormonal assay in blood (LH, FSH, sex hormones) for cases with precocious puberty.

*** Ultrasound scan is of great value in differentiating breast masses, e.g. a cyst from thelarche with normal tissue. Pelvic ultrasonography is indicated for precocious puberty in girls.

*** Fine-needle aspiration and biopsy are essential for evaluation of breast masses.

*** MRI or CT scan may demonstrate central nervous system abnormality in cases with precocious puberty.

*** Wrist X-ray for bone age to assess osseous maturation for cases of precocious puberty.

TOP TIPS

☑ Premature breast development (thelarche) is defined as an isolated breast enlargement in girls under the age of 7 years. Precocious puberty is defined as the presence of other puberty signs (pubic and/or axillary hair, growth spurt) under the age of 8 years in girls and under the age of 9 years in boys.

☑ Fibroadenoma is the most frequent breast tumour, seen frequently in adolescents, which is usually solitary and benign.

☑ Breast trauma is common often resulting from contact sport. Haematoma, contusion and fat necrosis may occur. The latter results from cystic changes or fibrosis within the breast.

☑ Painful engorgement of the breast (mastodynia) occurs physiologically in association with ovulatory cycles and pathologically in lactating mothers.

☑ In contrast to adults, mammography is not used in paediatrics because of the extremely low incidence of cancer, the risk of radiation and the dense breast tissue of adolescents obstructing adequate visualisation.

☑ The vast majority of breast masses can be diagnosed clinically or with the help of ultrasound scan. Occasionally, fine-needle aspiration biopsy is required.

☑ Any breast cyst that varies in size in relation to the menstrual cycle should be re-examined 2 weeks after the initial examination.

Red flags

- ◪ Breast buds (stage 2 of breast development), heralding puberty in girls, may be tender on palpation; this does not suggest inflammation.
- ◪ Although premature thelarche is a benign condition even if it starts as early as under 1 year of age, thorough examination is essential to ensure there are no signs of precocious puberty.
- ◪ Beware that a relapse of acute lymphoblastic leukaemia may present as a breast lump.
- ◪ Although malignant tumours are rare in children, their incidence is 2%–3% of all breast masses in adolescent girls. Early menarche in association with anovulatory cycles is a risk factor.
- ◪ A breast cancer is recognised by its rapid growth, which is hard and not freely mobile. Changes of the overlying skin including ulceration and nipple discharges are worrying signs.

NOTES:

NIPPLE DISCHARGE

The clinician overview

Unless the cause of nipple discharge is obvious (e.g. local inflammation or medication induced), this phenomenon must be carefully evaluated, the same as for adults. Although the condition is usually alarming for parents, fortunately its causes are usually benign in children. Discharge may be persistent or intermittent, scant or abundant, free-flowing or elicited by nipple stimulation, unilateral or bilateral. It is due to a variety of causes. In general, milky discharge, thick or not, suggests a benign condition (except galactorrhoea due to pituitary prolactinoma), while purulent discharge suggests infection, and serous or bloody discharge may suggest mastitis, duct ectasia, intraductal papilloma or cancer.

Possible diagnoses

INFANTS
Common
- ☑ Physiologic
- ☑ Acute mastitis
- ☑ Areola abscess
- ☑ Medication induced
- ☑ Mammary duct ectasia

Rare

CHILDREN
- ☑ Local stimulation
- ☑ Mammary duct ectasia
- ☑ Drugs (e.g. contraceptives)
- ☑ Pregnancy
- ☑ Prolactinoma (prolactin-secreting pituitary tumour)

- ☑ Breast infection (mastitis/abscess)
- ☑ Breast cancer
- ☑ Intraductal papilloma
- ☑ Fibroadenoma
- ☑ Hypothyroidism
- ☑ Fibrocystic breast disease
- ☑ Montgomery's tubercles
- ☑ Injury to the breast
- ☑ Idiopathic

Differential diagnosis at a glance

	Local stimulation	Mammary duct ectasia	Drugs	Pregnancy	Prolactinoma
Common in adolescents	Yes	Possible	Possible	Yes	Possible
Bilateral	Possible	Yes	Yes	Yes	No
May occur in boys	No	Yes	Yes	No	Yes
CNS symptoms (e.g. headache)	No	No	No	No	Yes
Needs full evaluation	No	Possible	No	No	Yes

Recommended investigations

***   Prolactin level to check for hyperprolactinaemia; TFT to check for hypothyroidism. Occasionally FSH, LH and TSH measurements are required.

***   Microscopic examination to confirm the galactorrhoea by finding the presence of fat globules; culture of the discharge is indicated for purulent discharge.

***   Pregnancy test to be considered for post-puberty girls if pregnancy is suspected.

***   Examination by ultrasound scan may establish the diagnosis of mammary duct ectasia by showing dilated ducts.

***   MRI of the brain once hyperprolactinaemia is confirmed, or if there are clinical features of cerebral lesion.

TOP TIPS

◪ Bilateral breast enlargement is very common in neonates, which results from circulating maternal hormones. Associated nipple discharge (witch's milk) should best be left alone as manipulation may cause mastitis.

◪ Galactorrhoea is a discharge of milk or milk-like secretion from the breast in the absence of parturition.

◪ Bilateral nipple discharge almost certainly excludes serious intra-mammary diseases, e.g. tumour.

◪ Remember that hypothyroidism is second after pituitary pathology in causing galactorrhoea. So TFT should be carried out for any obscure case of nipple discharge.

◪ Thorough history of any medication should be obtained. Medications that may cause galactorrhoea include metoclopramide, tricyclic antidepressants, phenothiazines, contraceptive pills.

◪ Another rare underlying disorder of galactorrhoea is hypothyroidism. TFT should be obtained in case of unclear aetiology.

◪ Breast cancer is extremely rare in young children. However, parents may seek medical consultation for fear of breast cancer. Their concerns should be addressed.

- Teenage pregnancy in the United Kingdom is the highest in Europe. Unless the cause is clear, a pregnancy test is indicated.
- Examination of the discharge assists in diagnosis: the secretion in benign conditions is usually milky thick or clear; infection is associated with purulent discharge, and in cancer it is usually serous or bloody.
- In galactorrhoea (spontaneous flow of milk), pituitary prolactinoma may be the underlying pathology; obtain urgently a serum prolactin level (abnormal if the level > 200 ng/mL) and consider head MRI.
- Prolactinoma is among the most common type of pituitary tumours. The level of prolactin correlates well with the tumour size.
- In any case of galactorrhoea, central nervous system examination should be performed, including visual examination, to exclude pituitary or hypothalamic tumour.
- Idiopathic galactorrhoea should not be diagnosed easily unless other possible underlying conditions have been eliminated by thorough history, examination and laboratory evaluation; it is a diagnosis of exclusion.
- Bloody nipple discharge may indicate mastitis or breast abscess; duct ectasia (obstruction of lactiferous ducts) also needs to be considered. The latter disorder may mimic breast cancer.

NOTES:

Ear

Earache (otalgia)

Ear discharge

Deafness/impaired hearing

Dizziness and vertigo

EARACHE (OTALGIA)

The clinician overview

Otalgia is one of the most common reasons for seeking medical attention. The pain usually arises from inflammation in the middle or external canal of the ear (intrinsic causes). Viruses such as adenovirus, RSV and influenza are the most common causes of otitis media (OM). Pseudomonas and staphylococci are the most common causes of otitis externa (OE). In infancy, the pain usually manifests as irritability, screaming and tenderness when the ear is rubbed or touched. In contrast to adults, referred pain from outside the ears (extrinsic causes) is common in paediatrics, occurring via five main sources: trigeminal nerve (sensory distribution of the face, teeth, gums); facial nerve (temporomandibular joint or Bell's palsy); glossopharyngeal nerve (tonsils, pharynx); vagus nerve (laryngopharynx or oesophagus) or via second and third cervical vertebrae (cervical spine). In all these cases patients have a normal otological examination.

Possible diagnoses

INFANTS
Common
- Infective OM
- Infective OE
- Trauma (cauliflower ear)
- Barotitis media (aerotitis)
- Infected eczematous dermatitis

Rare
- Furunculosis
- Acute cellulitis of the auricle

CHILDREN
- Infective OM
- Infective OE
- Referred pain (toothache, tonsillopharyngitis)
- Foreign body (FB) and trauma
- Barotitis media (during aviation)

- Myringitis (eardrum inflammation but without OM)
- Mastoiditis
- Trigeminal neuralgia
- Temporomandibular arthritis
- Ramsay Hunt Syndrome (herpes zoster oticus)
- Perichondritis/chondritis
- Cholesteatoma

- ◪ Exostoses and osteoma
- ◪ Impacted cerumen
- ◪ GO reflux
- ◪ Psychogenic

Differential diagnosis at a glance

	Infective OM	Infective OE	Referred pain	FB	Barotitis
Fever	Yes	Possible	Possible	No	No
Associated URTI	Yes	No	No	No	Possible
Abnormal eardrum	Yes	No	No	No	Yes
Being infant	Yes	Possible	Possible	No	Possible
Tender on touch	Possible	Yes	No	Yes	No

Recommended investigations

Laboratory tests are not necessary in the majority of children with otalgia
* FBC: leukocytosis > 15 000 may suggest bacterial infection, including occult infection.
*** Ear swab for culture in case of ear discharge.
*** X-ray and/or CT of the mastoid bone to confirm mastoiditis or sinusitis or cervical diseases.

TOP TIPS

- ◪ Mothers often seek medical consultation for fear of ear infection because their babies frequently touch their ears. In the absence of other symptoms, e.g. irritability or fever, this is harmless.
- ◪ Note that cerumen (wax) is a perfectly normal constituent of the ear canal; it becomes problematic only when it obstructs the view to the eardrum or causes hearing loss.
- ◪ When a child presents with otalgia in one ear, always examine the ear that does not hurt first.
- ◪ Otalgia of OE is characteristically aggravated by traction of the auricle and pressure on the tragus. A common and important cause is FB (20%–25% of all causes of otalgia referred to ENT specialist).
- ◪ While constant pain is usually otogenic, intermittent pain often suggests referred or psychogenic causes. The latter cause is suggested by, for example, the presence of emotional stress and absence from school.
- ◪ Note that the cartilaginous outer ear, containing one-third of the ear, is the site for furunculosis, while blunt trauma to the external ear, affecting the inner two-thirds, causes perichondritis and chondritis.
- ◪ Remember that severe or excruciating pain is likely to be otogenic (e.g. furunculosis,

myringitis) while mild to moderate pain is usually non-otogenic.

◪ Barotitis (symptoms of earache or discomfort, transient hearing loss and, rarely, bleeding) may occur during a sudden ambient pressure increase subsequent to descent or ascent of an aeroplane, or deep-sea diving in the presence of a dysfunctional Eustachian tube by an URTI.

◪ If symptoms of barotitis are felt, Valsalva's manoeuvre helps: take a good-sized breath, hold the nose and try to force air into the Eustachian tube by gently puffing out the cheeks with closed mouth.

◪ OM nowadays is most commonly caused by viral infections. Simple analgesic (paracetamol or ibuprofen) can provide relief. Antibiotics are often unnecessary. Do not give aspirin!

◪ Ramsay Hunt syndrome (auditory herpes zoster) usually presents with severe ear pain. Clues for this syndrome are vesicles on the pinna and in the external auditory canal in the distribution of the sensory branch of the facial nerve.

◪ Parents should be advised to be cautious about air travel if their child has an URTI or allergy as the relative negative pressure in the middle ear may result in retraction of the tympanic membrane, causing pain and possibly bleeding in the middle ear (barotitis).

Red flags

◪ In neonates, trauma to the pinna may present as haematoma with evolution to cauliflower ear. Immediate needle aspiration of the haematoma is necessary to prevent perichondritis, which can be refractory.

◪ The tympanic membrane of a crying baby is often red on inspection; do not misdiagnose OM.

◪ The presence of otalgia in the absence of otologic findings indicates the need for a thorough work-up to determine the source of referred pain.

◪ Beware that in Ramsay Hunt syndrome the associated hearing loss and facial palsy may be permanent (in about 50%).

◪ Remember that some topical otic preparations (neomycin, colistin, polymyxin) used to treat OE can cause contact dermatitis, which manifests as erythema, vesiculation and oedema.

NOTES:

EAR DISCHARGE

The clinician overview

Although otitis media (OM) is the most common cause of ear discharge, this diagnosis has become infrequent in recent years, mainly because of widespread vaccination, effective antibiotics and better living standards. Risk factors in neonates include nasotracheal intubation for more than 7 days, cleft palate and prematurity. Children are at high risk for OM and ear discharge if they are in a smoking environment, attend day care, have frequent colds, allergic rhinitis or adenoid hypertrophy. Pus from an infected OM or otitis externa (OE) needs to be differentiated from earwax (light, dark or orange-brown, normal odour) and water that entered the ear canal during showering or swimming.

Possible diagnoses

INFANTS
Common
- Discharge from passage through birth canal
- Suppurative OM
- Infective OE
- Haemorrhagic diathesis (disseminated intravascular coagulation)
- Seborrhoeic dermatitis

Rare
- Congenital cholesteatoma

CHILDREN
- Suppurative OM
- Infective OE
- Seborrhoeic dermatitis
- Otorrhoea from tympanostomy tube
- Trauma

- Acquired cholesteatoma
- Infected foreign body
- Otorrhoea (cerebrospinal fluid (CSF))
- Herpes zoster
- Mastoiditis
- Tumour (e.g. rhabdomyosarcoma, granuloma)

Differential diagnosis at a glance

	OM	OE	Seborrhoeic dermatitis	Otorrhoea	Trauma
Fever	Yes	Possible	No	Possible	No
Associated URTI	Yes	No	No	No	No
Purulent	Yes	Yes	No	Possible	No
Normal eardrum	No	Yes	Yes	Yes	Possible
Associated skin lesions	No	No	Yes	No	No

Recommended investigations

***   Culture of the infected discharge to identify the organisms.

**   CT scan or MRI if the symptom persists and no identifiable cause can be found.

TOP TIPS

- After an acute OM, about 40% of children develop otitis media with effusion (OME) that persists for a month and 10% have a persistent OME after 3 months.
- Following tympanostomy tube insertion for OME at least 50% of children develop otorrhoea through the tube while the tube is properly in place and patent.
- Besides a pus swab, the only other investigation necessary is audiological testing. Radiological investigations are usually required for complicated cases that should be referred.
- A pus swab for culture should be taken from the discharge and the ear canal cleaned. Ear toilet is very important. Frequent mopping of the ear canal using cotton pads is recommended; syringing of the ear is contraindicated and no instrument should be inserted into the ear canal blindly.
- OE, also called swimmer's ear, tends to recur in children who swim. An instillation of 2% acetic acid immediately after swimming is the most effective prevention. Children should not swim during and after an acute OE (until the infection is completely cleared) and the ears should be protected from water during bathing.

- The most serious complication of OM is intracranial suppurative infections including meningitis, subdural empyema and otogenic brain abscess.
- If otorrhoea persists despite adequate antibiotic cover, and if the source of discharge is pars flaccida (upper part of the tympanic membrane), cholesteatoma should be suspected.
- Clear discharge from the ear may be CSF resulting from basilar skull fractures. The CSF otorrhoea, along with facial palsy, is temporary. Fluid should be analysed to confirm it is CSF.
- Bloody discharge may follow a direct trauma; however, it is important to exclude a foreign object in the ear canal or, although rare, a cancer.
- A child with suppuration in the middle ear or mastoid is at risk of developing subdural or extradural abscess, meningitis, brain abscess.

NOTES:

DEAFNESS/IMPAIRED HEARING

The clinician overview

Hearing impairment is either sensorineural or conductive. The conductive hearing impairment is very common: at least half of preschool children have one or more episodes of otitis media with effusion (OME), which is often a cause of varying degrees of hearing impairment, usually mild (30–50 dB). The incidence of congenital sensorineural is approximately one per 1000 neonates, usually severe (50–70 dB) or profound (> 70 dB). High-risk factors for developing this type of hearing impairment are low gestation (< 32 weeks), prolonged jaundice, ototoxic drugs, hypoxic ischaemic encephalopathy, congenital infections (cytomegalovirus, rubella, syphilis) and neonatal meningitis.

Possible diagnoses

INFANTS
Common
- Congenital/genetic
- Drugs (ototoxic drugs)
- Low gestation (< 32 weeks)
- Prolonged jaundice
- Infection

Rare
- Waardenburg's syndrome
- Osteogenesis imperfecta
- Pendred's syndrome

CHILDREN
- OME (glue ear)
- Genetic
- Trauma (including acoustic trauma)
- Drugs (ototoxic drugs)
- Infection (e.g. following meningitis)

- Acoustic neuroma
- Osteopetrosis
- Histiocytosis
- Pendred's syndrome
- Osteogenesis imperfecta
- Lyme disease
- Waardenburg's syndrome
- Alport's syndrome
- Otosclerosis (autosomal dominant)

Differential diagnosis at a glance

	OME	Genetic	Trauma	Drugs	Infection
Severe/profound	No	Yes	Possible	Possible	Possible
Congenital	No	Yes	No	No	No
Likely onset in SCBU	No	No	No	Yes	Possible
Abnormal examination finding	Yes	No	Yes	No	No
Detected by screen	No	Yes	No	Possible	Possible

Recommended investigations

** Tympanogram if flat is likely to indicate significant effusion in the middle ear.

** Pure tone audiogram for more mature and cooperative children.

TOP TIPS

☑ Glue ear is caused by obstruction of the Eustachian tube, often by adenoids, so that air cannot enter the middle ear. As a result, fluid is produced, which affects the movement of the ossicles.

☑ As parents may not recognise mild or high-frequency hearing impairment and, as hearing impairment has a major impact on the child's development, screening testing during the neonatal period is strongly advocated (before 3 months of age).

☑ The most popular screening is evoked otoacoustic emissions (EOAE). Although EOAE testing is inexpensive and results are easy to interpret, it has a high failure rate for day 1 and 2 of life (about 40%). Those who fail the test must be evaluated further by auditory brainstem response (brainstem evoked response audiometry).

☑ Although most OME is transient, some children (e.g. those with Down syndrome, cleft palate) are at high risk of developing persistent effusion.

☑ Although the insertion of grommets for OME is effective in improving language acquisition, this effect lasts as long as the grommets are patent. Long-term benefits are not certain. Antibiotics, antihistamine, decongestants and steroids are usually ineffective.

☑ Usually OME has little influence on speech and language development.

☑ Beware the impact of high-frequency hearing loss on a child: they appear to hear well but are poor at understanding what is said – it is just a mumble of unclear sounds. Consonant sounds can only be heard faintly.

☑ When babies at risk of hearing loss are discharged from the SCBU, hearing and speech should be monitored closely. Parents and the SCBU should keep documentation on whether the child passed the screening test.

☑ Beware that congenital deafness due to congenital infection or genetic causes may deteriorate during the first 2 years of life and may escape neonatal screening testing.

- An 18-month-old child who has not said a single word with meaning or a 24-month-old child with a vocabulary of fewer than 10 words should be referred for audiologic assessment.
- When parents suspect their child's hearing is inadequate or delayed this must be taken seriously. A rapid referral to an audiological centre should be available in every part of the country.

Red flags

- Distraction hearing testing performed at the age of 6–9 months has more value if the technique follows standard guidelines. In practice, the test has low sensitivity and many cases of hearing impairment are missed.
- Any child with impaired speech development, recurrent ear infections or developmental or behavioural problems should have an audiological assessment.
- Beware that exposure to high-intensity sound (e.g. 80–100 dB in rock music) can cause temporary hearing loss. Sudden and very loud sound of more than 140 dB (e.g. gunfire, bombs) may cause permanent hearing loss after one exposure. Testing after such events might be important.
- Beware that some children considered 'slow' in learning might have high-frequency hearing loss. This impairs their ability to hear many high-pitched consonant sounds. Hearing aids are needed.
- A child with unilateral progressive deafness, vertigo and tinnitus should be suspected as having acoustic neuroma. Children with neurofibromatosis are at higher risk of developing this tumour.

NOTES:

DIZZINESS AND VERTIGO

The clinician overview

Dizziness is difficult to differentiate from vertigo in young children; therefore, the two conditions are joined in this section. Dizziness refers to a sensation of unsteadiness without the perception that the surroundings are rotating. Orthostatic hypotension is a prototype of this category. In true vertigo (such as vestibular neuritis), an older child complains of not only instability but also a feeling of spinning or turning. The underlying cause is somewhere in the equilibratory pathway (vestibule, semicircular canals, eighth nerve, vestibular nuclei in the brainstem and eyes). Fortunately, most causes of childhood vertigo are self-limiting. A young child with vertigo usually appears pale and frightened and/or suddenly falls to the ground, stumbles or is clumsy. Very often older children will describe a feeling of spinning or turning.

Possible diagnoses

INFANTS
Common
- Physiological (10–18 months of age)
- Benign paroxysmal vertigo (BPV)
- Drugs (e.g. sedative, antihistamine)
- Labyrinthitis (usually caused by viruses)
- Hypoglycaemia

Rare
- Cerebellar tumour

CHILDREN
- BPV
- Middle-ear and Eustachian disease
- Vestibular neuritis (VN)
- Orthostatic hypotension (not true vertigo)
- Labyrinthitis

- Trauma
- Migraine (basilar artery migraine)
- Hypoglycaemia
- Fistula between the middle and inner ear
- Vestibular neuritis (usually caused by viral infection)
- Ménière's disease (rare in children)
- Drugs (e.g. antidepressants, antihistamines, anticonvulsants)
- Epilepsy (temporal lobe epilepsy)
- Acoustic neuroma (about 6% of all intracranial tumours)

- Cerebellar tumour
- Cholesteatoma
- Mastoiditis
- Epidemic vertigo (caused by a virus, often following an upper respiratory tract infection)

Differential diagnosis at a glance

	BPV	Middle-ear and Eustachian disease	VN	Orthostatic hypotension	Labyrinthitis
True vertigo	Yes	Possible	Yes	No	Yes
Paroxysmal	Yes	No	Yes	No	Yes
Nystagmus	Yes	No	Yes	No	Yes
Fever	No	Yes	No	No	Possible
Hearing loss	No	Possible	No	No	Yes

Recommended investigations

** Blood sugar to confirm hypoglycaemia.

** Audiogram and tympanometry to assess the ear function and to distinguish labyrinthitis from VN.

*** EEG if there is a suspicion of epilepsy, such as loss of consciousness.

*** ECG if the cause of syncope is not clear and to exclude prolonged QT time.

** Ice-water caloric testing to confirm the abnormal vestibular function.

*** MRI or CT scan to exclude intracranial lesions, e.g. acoustic neuroma.

TOP TIPS

- Rough testing of the vestibular nerve is done by holding the child in arms and rotating them clockwise and anticlockwise. The normal eye deviation in the direction of rotation and nystagmus in the opposite direction is absent.
- Vertigo is often divided into peripheral vertigo and central vertigo. A referral to an otologist (who will deal with the peripheral part) and neurologist (who will deal with the central part) is often necessary.
- A clear distinction between BPV and migraine is absent. Many children with BPV will go on to develop migraine; vertigo occurs in about 50% of patients with basilar artery migraine.
- BPV occurs mainly in toddlers and manifests as sudden appearance of pallor, unsteadiness causing the child to fall, cries for help, clinging to their mother or refusal to walk. There is often vomiting and horizontal nystagmus. The episodes usually last up to 30 seconds. Attacks may recur in days or weeks
- Note that the onset of BPV usually occurs at the age of 2–8 years; however, it may occur in infancy. With time, attacks either cease or evolve into common migraine.
- In paediatrics the most common reason for dizziness is orthostatic hypotension, which manifests as feeling unsteady or fainting when getting up from sleep or from sitting for a long time.
- Remember that when labyrinthitis recurs, the diagnosis is often changed to Ménière's disease. Symptoms of both diseases are similar and overlap.
- The role of the clinician when seeing a child with vertigo is to exclude rare cases of a serious nature.

Red flags

- Any history of impaired or loss of consciousness in association with vertigo should alert the clinician that the attack could be epileptic (temporal lobe epilepsy).
- Unless the cause of the vertigo is clear (e.g. otitis media, BPV), close cooperation among different specialists (e.g. otologist, neurologist, sometimes ophthalmologist and psychiatrist) is essential to establish early diagnosis and management.
- Beware that although vasovagal syncope is usually benign in the majority of cases, atypical syncope may be due to arrhythmia. If so, referral to a paediatric cardiologist is indicated.
- Beware that, in addition to vertigo, children with acoustic neuroma often have nystagmus and unilateral deafness. Children with neurofibromatosis type 2 may develop this rare tumour.

NOTES:

Eye

Acutely red eye

Proptosis (exophthalmos)

Squint (strabismus)

Acute and transient loss of vision

Double vision (diplopia)

Eyelid disorders and ptosis

ACUTELY RED EYE

The clinician overview

Acutely red eye is common and caused by a variety of conditions including trauma such as a foreign body (FB) entering the eye, diseases of the conjunctive (conjunctivitis), cornea (keratitis), iris, ciliary body and choroid (uveitis), aqueous humour (glaucoma) and the sclera (scleritis and episcleritis). Clinicians should be able to diagnose most common eye diseases, which include allergic conjunctivitis (often seasonal with significant itching, runny nose, swollen lids and positive family history) and viral conjunctivitis (with its redness all over the conjunctive, watery discharge often beginning in one eye, usually caused by adenovirus). Bacterial conjunctivitis is commonly caused by chlamydia in neonates and by staphylococci in older children. It usually produces redness, maximal at the inferior conjunctiva and purulent discharge or keratitis with redness surrounding the cornea. Any eye redness in neonates or infants requires the exclusion of nasolacrimal duct obstruction and sub-conjunctival haemorrhage, which may result from injury, inflammation, severe straining (e.g. in mothers during delivery), sneezing or coughing. Referral to an ophthalmologist is indicated whenever the diagnosis is unclear.

Possible diagnoses

INFANTS
Common
- Lacrimal duct obstruction
- Chlamydia conjunctivitis
- Episceral haemorrhage during birth
- Chemical conjunctivitis (use of silver nitrate for prophylaxis)
- Bacterial conjunctivitis

Rare
- Gonococcal conjunctivitis
- Allergic conjunctivitis
- Dacryocystitis

CHILDREN

- Viral conjunctivitis
- Bacterial conjunctivitis
- Trauma (including FB)
- Allergic conjunctivitis
- Keratitis (e.g. herpetic keratitis, contact lens keratitis)

- Conjunctivitis associated with systemic diseases
- Acute uveitis
- Dacryocystitis
- Chemical conjunctivitis
- Epidemic keratoconjunctivitis (EKC)
- Haemorrhagic conjunctivitis
- Glaucoma

- Endophalmitis (a bacterial infection)
- Vernal conjunctivitis
- Syphilitic interstitial keratitis
- Haemorrhagic conjunctivitis (e.g. caused by picornavirus)
- Biotinidase deficiency (resulting in biotin deficiency)
- Cogan's syndrome (interstitial keratitis with hearing loss)
- Membranous and pseudomembranous conjunctivitis
- Chalazion and Hordeolum

Differential diagnosis at a glance

	Viral conjunctivitis	Bacterial conjunctivitis	Trauma	Allergic conjunctivitis	Keratitis
Seasonal	No	No	No	Yes	No
Unilateral	Possible	Possible	Yes	No	Possible
Impaired visual acuity	No	No	Possible	No	Yes
Overall redness	Yes	No	Possible	Yes	Possible
Severe itching	No	No	Possible	Yes	Possible

Recommended investigations

If the diagnosis of conjunctivitis in children is clear, laboratory testing, such as culture, is usually not necessary as conjunctivitis is common and harmless. Infection of the cornea by herpes virus produces branch-like (dendritic) lesions, which is demonstrated by fluorescein staining.

** FBC: leukocytosis for bacterial infection.

** ANA, rheumatoid factor (RhF) for children with rheumatoid arthritis.

*** Swab for purulent and severe discharge to exclude chlamydia or gonococcal infection.

*** Imaging of the orbit with MRI for any tumour such as rhabdomyosarcoma or in orbital cellulitis.

*** Tonometry to measure eye pressure for suspected glaucoma.

TOP TIPS

- Episcleral and retinal haemorrhages in neonates are common after vaginal delivery. Although these seem alarming to parents and clinicians, they are harmless and disappear within 2 weeks.

- Ophthalmia neonatorum refers to inflammation of the conjunctiva within the first month of life. Once principally caused by gonococcal infection, the most common cause is now chlamydia, staphylococci and chemical conjunctivitis caused by the topical antimicrobial agent, silver nitrate. The latter agent reduced the incidence of gonococcal ophthalmia from 10% to 0.3% in 1881.
- At birth, the nasolacrimal duct is often blocked. This resolves spontaneously in over 95% over the next few months, rarely delayed until the age of 1 year and very rarely needing surgery.
- Diagnosis of lacrimal duct obstruction is made by the history or by refluxing discharge with a pressure over the lacrimal sac.
- Measurement of visual acuity is needed for chronic cases, e.g. keratitis, not for conjunctivitis.
- Uveitis present with pain, lacrimation, photophobia and conjunctival hyperaemia. It occurs mainly in children with a mono-articular or pauci-articular form of rheumatoid arthritis.
- Children with glaucoma usually present with corneal irritation (tearing, photophobia), conjunctival infection and visual impairment. The most important sign is corneal enlargement.
- Remember that bilateral redness of the eyes often suggests viral or allergic conjunctivitis, while unilateral redness suggests FB. The latter one may need to be detected by everting the upper lid to check for concealed FB.
- Pain is not usually caused by conjunctivitis, but rather by uveitis, keratitis, glaucoma or scleritis.
- A child with red eyes and impaired vision is unlikely to have conjunctivitis. Keratitis is more likely. Ask whether there is a 'gritty sensation', which may occur with keratitis.

Red flags

- Gonococcal conjunctivitis presents in the first few days of life with a rapidly progressive profuse purulent discharge. The cornea is rapidly affected. Urgent treatment with antibiotics is needed.
- Conjunctivitis in neonates may be caused by STD acquired during vaginal delivery. Ensure you do not miss chlamydia or gonococcal infection.
- Ophthalmia neonatorum is a potentially blinding disease; it needs urgent diagnosis and treatment.
- Chlamydia is the most common cause of neonatal conjunctivitis in this country. Although it is often harmless, 10%–20% of infants experience chlamydial pneumonia, which is a serious disease. Therefore, infants should receive topical as well as systemic antibiotics.
- EKC is highly infectious, caused by adenovirus type 8. Hygienic measures, e.g. hand washing, are essential to prevent spread of the disease.
- Steroids should never be prescribed unless herpes infection is excluded. If diagnosis is not clear, referral to an ophthalmologist is indicated.
- Orbital cellulitis, presents as red and swollen eye, must be differentiated from rhabdomyosarcoma, which is a very aggressive malignancy of embryonic muscle tissue within the orbit. The tumour is often curable with radiation and radiotherapy.

NOTES:

PROPTOSIS (EXOPHTHALMOS)

The clinician overview

Proptosis, exophthalmos or protrusion of the eyes is a forward displacement of the eye, which may be caused by a congenital shallow orbit (craniofacial malformation such as oxycephaly, Crouzon's syndrome), trauma (orbital haemorrhage), inflammation (orbital cellulitis, abscess), vascular diseases (e.g. haemangioma, cavernous sinus thrombosis), central nervous system anomaly (encephalocele), endocrine (e.g. Graves' disease) and neoplasms (optic glioma, meningioma, metastatic neuroblastoma). Children with neurofibromatosis type 1 (NF-1) are at high risk of developing optic glioma and meningioma.

Possible diagnoses

INFANTS
Common
- Orbital capillary haemangioma
- Lymphangioma
- Lacrimal gland cyst/tumour
- Orbital teratoma
- Metastatic neuroblastoma

Rare
- Plexiform neurofibroma
- Congenital orbital varices
- Orbital encephalocele

CHILDREN

- Capillary haemangioma
- Orbital cellulitis
- Shallow orbit (e.g. Crouzon's syndrome)
- Tumour (optic nerve glioma, meningioma)
- Trauma (orbital haemorrhage)

- Deep dermoid cyst
- Plexiform neurofibroma
- Graves' disease (thyroid orbitopathy)
- Meningioma (involving sphenoid wing)
- Histiocytosis X
- Sarcoidosis
- Lymphangioma
- Neuroblastoma
- Non-specific orbital inflammatory syndrome
- Fibrous dysplasia
- Orbital encephalocele
- Wegener's granulomatosis
- Juvenile xanthogranuloma

Differential diagnosis at a glance

	Capillary haemangioma	Orbital cellulitis	Shallow orbit	Tumour	Trauma
Acute onset	No	Yes	No	Possible	Yes
Tenderness	No	Yes	No	Possible	Possible
Unilateral	Yes	Possible	No	Yes	Possible
Local inflammatory changes	No	Yes	No	Possible	Possible
Abnormal-shaped skull	No	No	Yes	No	No

Recommended investigations

**   FBC: leukocytosis suggests bacterial inflammation, differential count for suspected leukaemia.

***   TFTs for suspected hyperthyroidism.

***   Tumour markers in urine (VMA and HVA): elevated in neuroblastoma in 95%.

*   Skull X-ray for cranial tumour.

***   Renal ultrasound scan for metastatic neuroblastoma.

***   CT scan (most useful) for any suspected cranial tumour.

**   Aspiration cytology and biopsy occasionally required.

TOP TIPS

- Orbital capillary haemangioma is the most common orbital tumour in children, more often affecting the upper lid. Remember that the tumour has a rapid growth during the first 6 months of life and regresses spontaneously when the child reaches 4–6 years of age.
- The clinician faced with a child with proptosis should be able to do an ophthalmic examination, including assessment of visual acuity, ocular muscle movement, measuring of proptosis, pupillary size and reaction to light, fundi and performing systemic examination.
- Optic gliomas are very common with NF-1 (15%); they are usually benign and asymptomatic, and commonly present with visual disturbance. Unilateral glioma typically presents with afferent pupillary defect: a light source on the affected eye produces pupil dilatation (instead of constriction), while the unaffected eye produces bilateral pupil constriction.
- Proptosis caused by Graves' disease may occur in older children. Optic neuropathy, corneal problems and extraocular muscular involvement are far less common in children than in adults.
- Beware that a orbital cellulitis, often caused by paranasal sinusitis, first manifests as a red swelling of the lid. Prompt treatment with IV antibiotics at this stage dramatically improves the outcome.

- Neuroblastoma, the most common solid tumour of childhood, metastasises frequently into the orbit. The tumour may arise from the adrenals, cervical sympathetic chain or mediastinum.
- A proptotic eye not adequately protected by the lids is at risk of keratopathy, strabismus, diplopia, optic nerve atrophy and decreased visual acuity. Urgent management is required.
- Beware that prominent globe (e.g. caused by myopic enlargement) or eyelid retraction can be mistaken as proptosis.
- Orbital cellulitis must be recognised and treated promptly before serious complications occur, including extension of the infection into the cranial cavity causing meningitis, cavernous sinus thrombosis and epidural, subdural or brain abscess. Admission to hospital is urgently required.
- Be aware that a rapidly progressive swelling may suggest a malignant tumour such as rhabdomyosarcoma, metastatic neuroblastoma or Ewing's sarcoma.
- In a child who presents with Horner's syndrome with or without orbital ecchymoses, neuroblastoma has to be excluded.

NOTES:

SQUINT (STRABISMUS)

The clinician overview

Strabismus, misalignment of the eyes, is a common ophthalmic problem, affecting 4%–5% of children younger than 6 years of age. Strabismus is diagnosed clinically, which involves examination of the corneal light reflex and cover test. It may be transient or constant, manifest or latent. Because of different causes and treatments, it is important to divide strabismus into non-paralytic and paralytic. Non-paralytic strabismus includes inward deviation of the eyes (esophorias, commonly known as convergent or inward or crossed eyes), outward deviation of the eyes (known as exophorias, or divergent strabismus) and hyperdeviation (upward) and hypodeviation (downward) deviation of an eye. Paralytic strabismus involves palsy of the third, fourth or sixth cranial nerve. Strabismus may be congenital (or better termed 'infantile', as this allows inclusion of cases of strabismus that develop within the first few months of life) or acquired form. Of the most important and serious causes of the acquired form of strabismus is retinoblastoma.

Possible diagnoses

INFANTS
Common
- Pseudo-strabismus
- Congenital (infantile)
- Intermittent strabismus
- Paralytic strabismus
- Latent strabismus

Rare
- Möbius syndrome
- Duane syndrome
- Brown syndrome
- Parinaud syndrome

CHILDREN

- Pseudo-strabismus
- Congenital (infantile) non-paralytic strabismus
- Paralytic strabismus
- Accommodative strabismus
- Latent strabismus

- Migraine ophthalmoplegia
- Möbius syndrome (congenital bilateral facial weakness)
- Duane syndrome (congenital impaired eye motility)
- Parinaud syndrome (congenital weakness in vertical gaze)

☑ Brown syndrome (impaired elevation of the eye on adduction)

Differential diagnosis at a glance

	Pseudo-strabismus	Congenital non-paralytic strabismus	Paralytic strabismus	Accommodative strabismus	Latent strabismus
Normal corneal light	Yes	No	Yes	Yes	Possible
Associated with farsighted	No	No	No	Yes	No
Present under 6 months	Yes	Yes	Possible	No	Possible
Detected by cover test	No	Yes	No	No	Yes
Associated diplopia	No	Possible	Yes	No	No

Recommended investigations

***   Corneal light reflex for children who are not cooperative (under the age of 3 years). A light source is held between the examiner and the child at a distance of 25 cm. The light reflection is seen in the centre of the child's pupil in healthy eyes and in children with pseudo-strabismus.

***   Cover test for children who are cooperative. While the child looks at a distant object, the examiner covers each eye and watches for movement of the uncovered eye. This is followed by the rapid covering and uncovering of each eye. If there is any deviation, the eye rapidly moves as the cover moves to the other eye.

***   Orbital ultrasonography, CT scan for paralytic strabismus or retinoblastoma.

TOP TIPS

☑ Pseudo-strabismus is a common cause of referral to an ophthalmologist. It is usually caused by epicanthic folds or a broad flat nasal bridge. The normal alignment can be shown by the normal corneal light reflexes.

☑ An eye deviation that is present only when binocular vision is interrupted (by occlusion of one eye) is termed latent, while manifest deviation is present under binocular viewing of both eyes.

☑ Corneal light reflex is the most rapid and easily performed test to diagnose strabismus, particularly in children who are uncooperative.

☑ Accommodative strabismus, which usually manifests at 2–4 years of age, is a convergent strabismus occurring during accommodation (focusing) caused mainly by hyperopia (far-sighted).

- Up to the age of 6 months, intermittent strabismus is a normal developmental milestone, occurring particularly as outward deviation in about two-thirds of neonates. After the age of 6 months, any degree of strabismus needs to be evaluated.
- Note that an injury to the three ocular nerves (third, fourth and sixth) will cause strabismus, the angle of which will vary according to the direction of gaze.
- When patching is applied, be certain the parents fully understand the reason for the occlusion. Reward children when successful patching is maintained.

- Strabismus should never be ignored; it is never outgrown.
- In a child with any ocular disorder, including squints, assessment of the visual acuity is essential.
- Remember that the corneal light reflex is normal in paralytic strabismus.
- Untreated amblyopia (reduced visual acuity) results in permanent vision impairment.
- Beware that a fourth ocular nerve palsy causes a contralateral head tilt, i.e. a head tilt to the right caused by a left-sided nerve palsy and vice versa. Conversely, a sixth nerve palsy causes head tilting on the same side of the palsy. The reason for the tilt is to avoid diplopia.
- Retinoblastoma is most curable if diagnosed early; death is inevitable if untreated.
- Retinoblastoma, with an incidence of one in 20 000 births, is the most important cause of acquired strabismus. The tumour also presents with unilateral or bilateral leukocoria (a white pupil), orbital inflammation and/or a red eye reflex (cat eye).

NOTES:

ACUTE AND TRANSIENT LOSS OF VISION

The clinician overview

Visual loss may be acute or gradual, temporary or permanent. Acute visual loss is a frightening experience not only for children and their parents but also for the clinicians. Conditions causing acute visual loss in paediatrics are collectively uncommon (incidence estimated to be two–five cases per 10 000 births). It is either due to abnormalities within the ocular structure (cornea, lens, vitreous and retina) or neural visual pathways in the central nervous system (optic nerve, chiasm and cortical area). Visual loss within the eyes is easy to detect, e.g. corneal opacity, cataract or optic atrophy. Most causes of cortical visual loss occur in children with a neurodisability such as asphyxia at birth, in association with seizures, spasticity or hypotonia. Rarely, cortical visual loss occurs as an isolated neurological phenomenon. This section will discuss acute and transient visual loss only.

Possible diagnoses

INFANTS
Common
- Eye injury (birth trauma)
- Birth asphyxia (hypoxic-ischaemic encephalopathy)
- Hypoperfusion (anaemia, hypotension)
- Thrombosis (e.g. polycythaemia)
- Drugs (e.g. gentamicin)

Rare
- TORCH infection
- HIV infection
- Retinal detachment (e.g. from retinopathy of prematurity (ROP))
- Congenital varicella

CHILDREN
- Migraine
- Trauma (e.g. intracranial haemorrhage, eye injury)
- Infection (e.g. trachoma, meningitis, keratitis)
- Thromboembolic phenomenon
- Raised intracranial pressure (ICP) (optic glioma, posterior fossa tumour)

- Occipital lobe seizures
- Amaurosis fugax
- Macular degeneration
- Optic neuritis
- Acute glaucoma
- Stroke

- ☑ HIV infection
- ☑ Retinal migraine, artery or venous occlusion
- ☑ Collagen diseases (e.g. rheumatoid arthritis)
- ☑ Conversion symptom (hysteria)
- ☑ Cortical blindness
- ☑ Familial transient visual loss
- ☑ Postprandial transient visual loss (after heavy meal)
- ☑ Unexplained

Differential diagnosis at a glance

	Migraine	Trauma	Infection	Thromboembolic phenomenon	Raised ICP
Sudden onset	Yes	Yes	Yes	Yes	Possible
Progressive	No	Possible	Possible	Possible	Yes
Recurrent	Yes	Possible	Possible	Possible	No
Lasts < I hour	Yes	Possible	No	Possible	No
Monocular	Possible	Possible	Possible	Yes	Possible

Recommended investigations

**   TORCH screening test (IgM for cytomegalovirus, herpes simplex, rubella), urine for rubella virus isolation.

***   HIV DNA detected by polymerase chain reaction.

***   Orbital ultrasonography and CT scan of the eye and head for suspected tumour.

***   EEG for cases with seizures.

*   Electrophysiological testing with electroretinography for retinal causes of visual loss.

TOP TIPS

- Eye examination is an essential part of neonatal examination, including using the ophthalmoscope held at a distance of 20–25 cm to look for the red reflex. Fundoscopy is usually unnecessary.
- Although children with eye problems are often referred to ophthalmologists, clinicians should be able to perform certain eye examinations. These include examination of the visual fields (looking for the wiggly fingers), perform cornea light reflex, cover tests, fundoscopy. Visual acuity is tested by the child's ability to fixate and follow an object (brightly coloured toy).
- Detection of visual loss is essential because of availability of cure and for genetic implication (e.g. cataract, ROP, glaucoma and retinoblastoma).
- The most common cause for transient visual loss in children occurs during a visual aura of a classic migraine. Aura is defined by the International Headache Society as a recurrent disorder that develops over 5–29 minutes and lasts for < 1 hour.
- Transient monocular visual loss lasting 1–5 minutes is usually referred to as amaurosis fugax resulting from cerebral ischaemia (seizure, stroke). While migraine aura may present with flashes of light (photopsia), amaurosis fugax presents as blackout of vision or a curtain across the vision.
- In ophthalmology, more than in any other specialty, observation is the most important technique to detect abnormalities. Get the child interested in visual toys and games such as a bright-red object or the light source of a torch.
- Some systemically administered medications, e.g. steroids, may cause cataract. Steroids may also cause glaucoma.

- Beware that a child with leukocoria, a white pupil, has a major clinical implication: the likely cause is either retinoblastoma or cataract. Untreated or with delayed treatment, the retinoblastoma will lead to death, cataract to permanent vision loss.
- Remember a few important conditions causing sudden loss of vision: migraine or amaurosis fugax, thromboembolic events may occur in predisposed conditions such as polycythaemia, sickle-cell anaemia, homocystinuria.
- Occipital seizures (such as benign partial epilepsy with occipital paroxysm) are not rare; visual symptoms are prominent and include amaurosis, multi-coloured illusions or hallucinations and eye deviation, followed by hemiclonic seizures or automatisms. EEG is usually diagnostic.
- While papilloedema is a cardinal sign of increased ICP, in infants, separation of the cranial sutures and bulging of the anterior fontanel decompresses the ICP; papilloedema may not occur.

NOTES:

DOUBLE VISION (DIPLOPIA)

The clinician overview

Diplopia, simultaneous perception of two images of a single object, is less common in children than in adults because of the lower incidence of strokes and other intracranial lesions. The most common cause of diplopia in children is misalignment of the visual axes occurring particularly in disorders affecting the cranial nerves (third, fourth and sixth) innervating the six ocular muscles. Other causes involve mechanical interference with ocular motion or disorder of neuromuscular transmission. Diplopia is either binocular (true diplopia) or monocular. The latter is caused by abnormality in the cornea (e.g. severe astigmatism = irregular curvature), in the lens (e.g. cataract, dislocated lens) or in the vitreous humour (e.g. vitreous cysts). Diplopia is often the first manifestation of many systemic muscular or neurologic disorders, some of which are of a serious nature. Therefore, prompt evaluation is usually required. A detailed history and examination will make it possible to determine which muscles and ocular nerves are affected and what is the likely cause. Although diplopia does occur in infants, they do not usually present with diplopia and therefore the causes in infants are not included in this section.

Possible diagnoses

INFANTS
Common

CHILDREN

- Physiological
- Strabismus (particularly paralytic)
- Post-surgery for refractive errors
- Increased intracranial pressure (ICP)
- Myasthenia gravis (MG)

Rare

- Trauma
- Drugs (e.g. antiepileptics)
- Ophthalmoplegic migraine
- Thyroid ophthalmopathy
- Retinoblastoma
- Conversion symptom (hysteria)
- Basilar artery migraine
- Möbius syndrome

◪ Stroke
◪ Sarcoidosis

Differential diagnosis at a glance

	Physiological	Strabismus	Post-surgery	Increased ICP	MG
Detected by corneal light reflex	No	Yes	Yes	Yes	Possible
Present when fatigued	No	Possible	Possible	No	Yes
Associated vomiting, headache	No	No	No	Yes	No
Normal eyes	Yes	No	No	No	Yes
Ptosis	No	Possible	Possible	Possible	Yes

Recommended investigations

** Urine for sodium nitropruside test for suspected cases of homocystinuria (lens dislocation).

*** IV injection of short-acting edrophonium (Tensilon) to reverse the symptoms of MG.

*** Anti-acetylcholine antibodies in plasma for suspected MG.

*** TFTs for suspected cases of hyperthyroidism.

*** A chest X-ray for suggested cases of sarcoidosis to show bilateral hilar lymphadenopathy.

*** MRI of the head may show tumour, area of infarction or even arterial aneurysm.

*** Electromyogram (EMG) may be diagnostic in cases of MG.

TOP TIPS

◪ Differentiating monocular from binocular diplopia is simple: covering each eye will correct diplopia in binocular while diplopia persists in the monocular.

◪ Ophthalmoplegic migraine presents as third-nerve palsy ipsilateral to the hemicranial of the headache due to vasoconstriction during the attack to this nerve.

◪ Although the diagnosis of which ocular muscles are affected is fairly easy, a final diagnosis is unlikely to be reached at primary setting. Referral to an ophthalmologist is usually required.

◪ When a child presents with diplopia and ptosis, third-nerve palsy is likely. However, Horner's syndrome is another possibility. Small pupil and reduced sweating on the affected side will help to differentiate both conditions.

Red flags

- ☑ Diplopia may be the first complaint in children with a dislocated lens. This occurs in conditions such as Marfan's syndrome (excessive height, dilated aortic route) or homocystinuria (malar flush, neurodisability, thromboembolic events).
- ☑ The most common cause of diplopia is strabismus. However, the brain of a young child learns how to suppress the image of the weaker, misaligned eye. Therefore, diplopia is usually not the presenting complaint in young age.
- ☑ Any diplopia warrants prompt evaluation; it may signal a serious intracranial disease.
- ☑ Although diplopia is a common symptom in posterior fossa tumour, children rarely complain of it, as they are able to suppress the image of the affected eye. Instead, head tilting may occur as this position is an attempt to align the two images.
- ☑ Beware that fourth-nerve palsy typically presents with head tilting opposite to the affected eye, while sixth-nerve palsy tilts toward the palsied nerve.
- ☑ A typical basilar artery migraine (e.g. diplopia, vertigo, ataxia and headache) should be differentiated from intracranial tumour. An urgent CT scan or MRI is often needed, particularly if it is the first episode.
- ☑ Remember that the sixth nerve has a long intracranial course so it is susceptible to damage from cranial tumour. Beware that an acquired sixth-nerve palsy is usually an ominous sign requiring attention.
- ☑ Adolescents with hysteria may present with diplopia; this diagnosis should be one of exclusion.

NOTES:

EYELID DISORDERS AND PTOSIS

The clinician overview

Eyelid disorders are exceedingly common in children and range from benign, self-resolving to serious malignant or metastatic processes. Although the majority of these disorders are dealt with by ophthalmologists, this section will only stress those disorders that are important to the clinicians in relation to associated systemic diseases. For example, an acquired ptosis may be due to third-nerve palsy, caused by myasthenia gravis, myotonic dystrophy, botulism or Horner's syndrome. Therefore, the diagnosis of any eyelid abnormality requires thorough systemic examination and sometimes investigations to exclude systemic diseases.

Possible diagnoses

INFANTS
Common
- Coloboma
- Congenital ptosis
- Congenital ectropion
- Tumour (haemangioma, dermoid cyst)
- Epicanthic folds

Rare
- Congenital Horner's syndrome
- Congenital entropion
- Congenital muscular dystrophy

CHILDREN
- Epicanthic folds
- Coloboma (may be associated with Goldenhar syndrome)
- Acquired ptosis
- Tumour/cyst (e.g. haemangioma, cyst; mechanical ptosis)
- Acute blepharitis

- Acquired Horner's syndrome
- Meibomian cyst
- Chalazion (inflammation of the meibomian cyst)
- Myasthenia gravis (MG)
- Myotonic muscular dystrophy (Steinert disease)
- Muscular dystrophy (facioscapulohumeral type)
- Marcus Gunn jaw-winking phenomenon
- Sparse or absent eyebrows (ectodermal dysplasia, alopecia)

- ☑ Lash abnormalities
- ☑ Eyebrow abnormalities

Differential diagnosis at a glance

	Epicanthic folds	Coloboma	Acquired ptosis	Tumour/cyst	Acute blepharitis
Congenital	Yes	Yes	Possible	Possible	No
Bilateral	Yes	Possible	Possible	No	Possible
Affecting lid margins	No	Possible	No	No	Yes
Improve with age	Yes	No	No	No	Possible
Lid lag on downgaze	No	No	Yes	Possible	Possible

Recommended investigations

***   CPK in blood for muscular diseases.

***   Anti-acetylcholine antibodies in plasma for suspected MG.

**   Serum and/or stool for botulin toxin for suspected botulism.

***   A chest X-ray in cases of myasthenia gravis for evidence of enlarged thymus and thymoma.

**   ECG for cases of muscular dystrophy and myopathies.

***   CT scan of the anterior mediastinum to assess the thymus for the presence of possible thymoma.

***   Electromyogram (EMG) may be diagnostic in cases of MG, myotonic dystrophy.

TOP TIPS

- Epicanthic folds are folds across the inner corner of the eyes (canthus), usually from the upper lids. They are present in most infants and young children and become less apparent later, coinciding with peaking of the nasal bridge. If they are prominent, they give the impression of pseudo-strabismus.
- Not all small palpebral apertures are caused by ptosis; telecanthus (increased width between the medial canthi) and epicanthus inversus (epicanthic folds originating from the lower lid) can be the cause. The latter may be inherited as autosomal dominant; affected females are often infertile.
- While congenital ptosis is usually due to dystrophic levator muscle, acquired ptosis may occur in association with systemic disorders such as MG or myotonic dystrophy.
- In Marcus Gunn jaw-winking (5% of all cases with ptosis), the upper lid rises as the jaw opens. This is caused by synkinesis between the third and fifth cranial nerves.
- Eyebrow abnormalities include sparse or absent eyebrows (e.g. alopecia, ectodermal dysplasia) and eyebrows joining together medially (Waardenburg's syndrome, Cornelia de Lang syndrome).
- Although epicanthic folds are present in most healthy young children, they are often a cause of referral to ophthalmologists because of 'squint' appearance (pseudo-strabismus). Remember that occasionally they can be associated with syndromes and various chromosomal abnormalities.
- Children with ptosis should be referred for ophthalmic opinion and surgery if they have abnormal head posture, amblyopia, abnormal visual field and is cosmetically unacceptable.
- Beware that children with ptosis commonly raise the eyebrows or lift the chin in an attempt to maintain binocular vision.

Red flags

- While the congenital Horner's syndrome may be associated with vertebral anomalies, an acquired one may be the first presenting of mediastinal tumour such as neuroblastoma.
- Beware that entropion (inward-turning of the lid margin and lashes, trichiasis) often presents with irritability and can cause corneal damage. Urgent consultation with an ophthalmologist is required. Larsen's syndrome (entropion, multiple joint dislocations, cleft palate and neurodisability) has to be excluded.
- Patients with ectropion (outward-turning of the lid margin) are at risk of exposure keratopathy, overflow of tears and conjunctivitis. This may occur in association with facial palsy resulting from weakness of the orbicularis muscle. Again, urgent ophthalmic consultation is required.
- When an edrophonium (Tensilon) test is carried out to confirm MG, facility for cardiopulmonary resuscitation must be available. Prior to the test, the ptosis and strabismus are measured.

NOTES:

Face

Facial swelling

Facial rash

Acute facial pain

Facial weakness

FACIAL SWELLING

The clinician overview

Facial swelling is a common clinical paediatric problem. The term refers to an enlargement of any area of the face, including the eyes, nose, mouth, forehead, cheeks and chin. Swelling is usually caused by an abnormal build-up of fluid in the face, oedema, which is the most common cause of facial swelling. Oedema is either generalised – caused by systemic diseases such as nephrotic syndrome (NS), glomerulonephritis (GN), congestive cardiac failure (CCF), acute and chronic renal failure (ARF and CRF), hypoproteinaemia, agammaglobulinaemia – or localised – caused by allergy such as angioneurotic oedema or bee sting. Genuine oedema needs to be differentiated from 'puffy face' often found in association with obesity, hypothyroidism and Cushing's syndrome (CS). Facial masses are the second most common causes of facial swelling.

Possible diagnoses

INFANTS
Common
- ☑ Oedema (acute illness, excess IV fluid)
- ☑ Electrolyte imbalance (e.g. prematurity)
- ☑ ARF
- ☑ CCF
- ☑ Lymphoedema

Rare
- ☑ Haemangioma
- ☑ Parotid swelling (e.g. bacterial infection)

CHILDREN
- ☑ Dental abscess
- ☑ Haemangioma
- ☑ Obesity
- ☑ Allergy (angioneurotic oedema, bee sting)
- ☑ Generalised oedema (NS, hypogammaglobulinaemia)

- ☑ Parotid disease (mumps, parotid tumour, duct stone)
- ☑ Sinusitis
- ☑ Midline or nasal dermoid cyst
- ☑ Lymphoedema, lymphangioma
- ☑ Hypothyroidism
- ☑ Subcutaneous emphysema
- ☑ Trichinosis
- ☑ Cushing's syndrome (CS)
- ☑ CRF

- ◪ Superior vena cava obstruction
- ◪ Sarcoma (rhabdomyosarcoma, Ewing's sarcoma)
- ◪ Kimura's disease
- ◪ Metastatic neuroblastoma
- ◪ Fibrous dysplasia

Differential diagnosis at a glance

	Dental abscess	Haemangioma	Obesity	Allergy	Generalised oedema
Pitting	No	No	No	Possible	Yes
Associated pain	Yes	No	No	Possible	No
Unilateral	Yes	Yes	No	Possible	No
Associated itching	No	No	No	Yes	Possible
Swelling elsewhere	No	No	Yes	Possible	Yes

Recommended investigations

***   24-hour urine collection for protein in NS or GN, and for free cortisol measurement for CS.

***   Blood for serum albumin, triglyceride in suspected NS.

***   Renal function tests and U&E to determine ARF and CRF.

**   Blood for RAST or skin prick test in case of allergy.

***   Blood for dexamethasone suppression test for Cushing's syndrome.

***   Chest X-ray, ECG and echocardiography to diagnose the cause of CCF.

**   Ultrasound scan is useful for suspected facial tumour such as parotid tumour.

***   CT scan or MRI for sinusitis and underlying tumours.

***   Sialography to demonstrate salivary duct stone or inflammatory duct disease.

***   Percutaneous needle biopsy for tumour.

TOP TIPS

- A premature infant is at high risk of developing generalised oedema, including facial oedema, because of low glomerular infiltration rate and inability to handle water and solute loads.
- Dental abscess is the result of bacterial infection of the dental pulp (periapical abscess) or the gum (periodontal abscess).
- Angio-oedema (or angioneurotic oedema) is very similar to urticaria except it affects the deeper layers of subcutaneous and mucous tissues. Its intense pruritis and redness differentiates it from generalised oedema caused, for example, by hypoproteinaemia.
- Beware that the parotid gland can only be felt when it is enlarged. Swelling is seen as a bulge in front of the ear displacing the tragus.
- Facial oedema in developing countries may be due to protein malnutrition, while in developed countries NS, CCF and allergy are the usual causes.
- Lymphoedema, present as non-pitting oedema of the face, is either congenital (e.g. Milroy's disease, Turner's syndrome in girls, Noonan's syndrome in boys) or acquired following removal of lymph nodes for biopsy or radiation therapy for cancer; rarely it is caused by filariasis infection.
- Remember that an acute dental abscess may be painless and presents as fever, chills and pyrexia of unknown origin (PUO). Dental abscess needs to be excluded in any case of PUO.
- Facial swelling in association with pain and tenderness over the bones overlying the sinuses may indicate sinusitis, orbital cellulitis or cavernous sinus thrombosis.

Red flags

- Be aware that a rapidly progressive swelling may suggest a malignant tumour such as rhabdomyosarcoma or Ewing's sarcoma, while slowly progressive facial swelling is often caused by less serious conditions such as fibrous dysplasia, haemangioma or neurofibroma.
- Facial swelling may be caused by superior vena cava obstruction, which manifests as swollen face especially around the eyes, distended neck and prominent chest veins. Any condition predisposing to thrombosis (e.g. NS, sickle-cell anaemia) may cause such an obstruction.
- If a child presents with swelling of the glabellar area, then encephalocele, nasal glioma or midline or nasal dermoid cyst should be excluded. Although dermoid cyst is always congenital, it usually begins to enlarge in the first few years of age. Cases of encephaloceles have a patent intracranial connection; 25% of cases of dermoid cyst have intracranial connection.

NOTES:

FACIAL RASH

The clinician overview

A child's skin is more reactive than an adult's. For example, vesiculobullous eruptions are more common in children, and many systemic diseases present with cutaneous manifestations. In addition, the appearance of macules or patches does not commonly remain static, and acute eruption can change rapidly to become elevated (maculopapular) or blistering (maculovesicular). Facial rash in this section is classified according to a simple practical approach based on the morphological appearance of the rash:

> Macule (< 1 cm) and patch (> 1 cm): defined as alteration of skin colour but no elevation is felt.
> Papule (< 1 cm), nodule (> 1 cm) and tumour (> nodule): defined as palpable, solid lesions.
> Vesicle (< 1 cm) and bulla (> 1 cm): defined as fluid-filled, raised lesions.
> Purpura, extravasation of blood, is with petechiae (pinpoint) or ecchymoses (patches). Eruptions are often a mixture of lesions such as maculopapular, papulovesicular or vesiculobullous.

(Vascular and pigmented birthmarks are not included in this section; *see* Skin chapter)

Possible diagnoses

INFANTS
Common
- Papulovesicular (e.g. atopic dermatitis)
- Macules or patches (e.g. viral infectious diseases)
- Patch (salmon patch)
- Papulo-pustular (e.g. erythema toxicum)
- Papules (e.g. seborrhoeic dermatitis (SD))

CHILDREN
- Macules/patches (e.g. viral infections, allergy)
- Papules (e.g. SD, insect bites)
- Vesiculo-pustulous (e.g. non-bullous impetigo)
- Purpuric (e.g. meningococcaemia, thrombocytopenia)
- Papulovesicular (e.g. atopic dermatitis)

Rare

- ☑ Bullae (e.g. bullous impetigo)
- ☑ Vesiculo-bullous (herpes infections)

- ☑ Bullae (epidermolysis bullousa, bullous impetigo)
- ☑ Erythematous-bullous-vasculitic (systemic lupus erythematosus)
- ☑ Papulo-pustulo-nodular (acne)
- ☑ Vesiculo-bullous (poison, herpes infections, bullous impetigo, staphylococcal scalded skin syndrome)
- ☑ Papule-plagues (lichen planus)
- ☑ Patch, periorbital, violaceous (dermatomyositis)
- ☑ Papulosquamous (psoriasis, pityriasis rosea)
- ☑ Vesicles, linear (poison ivy contact dermatitis)
- ☑ Papules with burrows (scabies)

Differential diagnosis at a glance

	Macules/patches (e.g. viral infectious diseases)	Papules (e.g. SD)	Vesiculo-pustules (e.g. impetigo)	Purpuric (e.g. meningo-coccaemia)	Papulovesicular (e.g. atopic dermatitis)
Itching	Possible	No	Possible	No	Yes
Associated with fever	Yes	No	No	Yes	No
Rash elsewhere	Yes	Possible	No	Yes	Possible
May last for months	No	Yes	Possible	No	Yes
Respond to antibiotics	No	No	Yes	Yes	No

Recommended investigations

** FBC: leukopenia in some viral diseases, e.g. measles, leukocytosis, e.g. HHV-6 and bacterial infections, anaemia in systemic lupus erythematosus and low platelets in thrombocytopenia purpura.

** CRP: high in bacterial diseases, e.g. meningococcal disease.

*** BC for suspected cases of meningococcaemia.

** Auto-antibodies, ANA, double-stranded DNA in systemic lupus erythematosus and dermatomyositis.

*** Muscle enzymes (e.g. creatine phosphokinase), MRI and muscle biopsy for dermatomyositis.

TOP TIPS

- In contrast to atopic dermatitis (AD), SD often appears within the first month of life, disappears when the child is aged 1–2 years, and is usually non-pruritic.
- Most acute skin eruptions are non-pruritic. Among those rashes causing intense pruritis are urticaria, atopic dermatitis and lichen planus.
- Pruritis from any cause is always worse at night. The warmth of bedclothes causes vasodilatation in the skin, which worsens the itching. Ask parents how well their child sleeps at night.
- AD should be diagnosed with strict clinical criteria using major criteria (e.g. family or personal history of atopy, typical facial or extensor lesions) and minor criteria (elevated IgE, xerosis, susceptibility to infection).
- Urticaria (mostly caused by drugs, food or viruses) is often confused with erythema multiforme. The latter produces typical iris or target lesions and mucosal involvement is common.
- Although drugs can cause a variety of cutaneous morphologies, the most common drug-induced rashes are urticaria, erythema multiforme and maculopapular eruptions.
- Remember to examine the buccal mucosa in any child presenting with a rash. Examples include reticulate, white plagues in lichen planus and vesiculo-bullous in erythema multiforme.
- When children present with pruritic skin eruption, treating the pruritis is more important than the rash.
- Beware that rash due to sunburn may occur in cloudy weather without sun exposure.

Red flags

- Although purpura is the most common rash of meningococcal disease, other rashes include maculopapular, pustular and bullous lesions.
- Children with AD are at risk of serious complication with herpes simplex virus, eczema herpeticum, which can be fatal. Intravenous acyclovir is the mainstay of treatment.
- Beware that in children with cold urticaria, pruritic or painful rash appears on exposure to cold and is confined to the exposed parts of the body. Swimming in cold water is dangerous and can be fatal.

NOTES:

ACUTE FACIAL PAIN

The clinician overview

Facial pain, like any other pain, is an unpleasant sensory and emotional experience, and carries the risk of actual or potential tissue damage. The term is used to describe, on looking at the face, facial pain that may or may not have an obvious cause. Facial trauma caused by an accident is excluded, as there is a clear cause of the pain. Facial pain has a long list of disorders caused by an inflammation, vascular changes, an infection or tumour. Assessing facial pain and localising the source of the pain in children can be difficult, particularly in infants and young children. Nevertheless, diagnosis is usually possible by taking a good history and using pain assessment techniques classified as self-reporting, behavioural observation (such as facial expression, crying, forceful closure of the eyes) and physiologic measures (such as tachycardia, pupil dilatation).

Possible diagnoses

INFANTS
Common
- Otitis media
- Pharyngitis
- Facial osteomyelitis

CHILDREN

- Headaches (e.g. migraine, particularly cluster pain)
- Sinusitis
- Dental abscess
- Trigeminal neuralgia
- Tumour (benign or malignant)

Rare
- Facial osteomyelitis

- Temporomandibular joint dysfunction
- Glaucoma
- Atypical facial pain
- HIV infection
- Facial osteomyelitis (maxillary or mandibular)
- Herpes zoster (pre-rash appearance)
- Parotid gland
- Post-herpetic neuralgia (PHN)
- Tic douloureux
- Temporal arteritis

Differential diagnosis at a glance

	Headaches	Sinusitis	Dental abscess	Trigeminal neuralgia	Tumour
Fever	No	Possible	Possible	No	No
Associated swelling	No	Possible	Possible	No	Possible
Tenderness	Possible	Yes	Yes	No	Possible
Worse on bending	No	Yes	Yes	No	No
Associated vomiting/ nausea	Yes	Possible	No	Possible	Possible

Recommended investigations

**   FBC: raised WBC count in inflammatory conditions.

**   CRP and ESR: raised in infections, malignancy and temporal arteritis.

**   X-ray of the face may show opacification of the sinus or mastoid area.

**   Dental X-ray if a dental abscess is suspected.

***   CT/MRI scan, which is more specific than an X-ray in diagnosing sinusitis or facial tumour.

**   Sialography in suspected cases of parotid duct stone.

**   Fine-needle biopsy for suspected facial tumour confirmed by CT or MRI scan.

**   Tonometry: if glaucoma is suspected.

TOP TIPS

- In contrast to presentation of adolescents and adults with sinusitis (headaches, facial pain, tenderness, facial oedema), symptoms of sinusitis in pre-adolescent children are persistence of symptoms of upper respiratory tract infection, nasal discharge and cough. Cough is typically worse when lying down.
- Idiopathic facial pain is a deep and poorly localised pain that is present daily and persists most of the day. It is a diagnosis of exclusion, including cranial neuralgias. There is no sensory loss.
- PHN is defined as pain persisting for more than 3 months after the onset of herpes zoster rash. Up to 50% of older people are estimated to develop PHN following shingles.
- In managing pain, remember the stepwise approach, published by the World Health Organization, to escalating therapy from weak analgesics (e.g. paracetamol or NSAIDs) to strong ones (e.g. morphine).
- Although pressing over the area of sinuses is the best direct method of examination, beware that the child might find any pressure on the face to be painful.
- Remember that neuropathic pain (e.g. trigeminal neuralgia, HIV infection) is notoriously difficult to treat with opioids. Antidepressants (e.g. imipramine) and anticonvulsants (e.g. carbamazepine) are often effective.

- Beware that sinuses do not become potential infection sites in early childhood because they are not developed. Frontal sinuses, for example, are developed at 4–7 years of age.
- Headaches may be the underlying disorder of facial pain. Remember that the three important causes are migraine (usually throbbing), tension headaches (usually 'pressing') and tumour with increased intracranial pressure (may produce throbbing, pressing or sharp pain).

Red flags

- While the main site for neonatal facial osteomyelitis is in the area of maxillary bone and pre-maxillary suture, the mandible is the usual location in older children. In both locations, children present with swelling, fever (rare in neonates), pain and redness of skin and oral mucosa.

NOTES:

FACIAL WEAKNESS

The clinician overview

Facial weakness may be congenital or acquired, idiopathic or caused by infection, inflammation, trauma, tumour or vascular event. The most common cause of congenital facial weakness is trauma during delivery. The most common cause of acquired weakness is Bell's palsy, an isolated lower motor neuron lesion of the seventh nerve. As a rule, children with facial weakness have better prognosis than adults. Facial weakness should be differentiated from facial asymmetry, which may result from underdevelopment of the muscle controlling the lip, excessive moulding of the cranium or face presentation during delivery, or in older children with hemihypertrophy.

Possible diagnoses

INFANTS
Common
- Birth injury (e.g. forceps delivery)
- Infection (otitis media (OM), mastoiditis)
- Congenital myopathies (e.g. nemaline)
- Möbius syndrome
- Agenesis of depressor angularis oris muscle

Rare
- Transient myasthenia gravis
- CHARGE association
- Bell's palsy

CHILDREN

- Bell's palsy
- Infection (Lyme disease, OM, meningitis, herpes zoster)
- Myopathies (myotonic dystrophy)
- Möbius syndrome
- Myasthenia gravis

- Agenesis of the depressor angularis oris muscle
- CHARGE association
- CANOMAD syndrome
- Neuro-sarcoidosis

Differential diagnosis at a glance

	Bell's palsy	Infection	Myopathies	Möbius syndrome	Myasthenia gravis
Rapid onset	Yes	Yes	No	No	Possible
Bilateral	No	No	Possible	Possible	Possible
Confined to the seventh nerve	Yes	Possible	No	No	No
Recovery likely	Yes	Yes	No	No	Possible
Other cranial involvement	No	Possible	Possible	Yes	Yes

Recommended investigations

***   Anti-acetylcholine Abs for myasthenia.

***   Edrophonium test (0.2 mg/kg IV) in myasthenia; if positive, ptosis will improve within seconds.

***   EMG: more specifically diagnostic than a muscle biopsy in myasthenia gravis.

***   Neuroimaging: for cases not recovering.

**   Nerve conduction studies.

*   Muscle biopsy has limited value in myasthenia.

TOP TIPS

☑ Unilateral facial weakness due to forceps delivery has an almost 100% recovery rate, while the recovery rate of older children with the acquired form of Bell's palsy is 80%–90%.

☑ Möbius syndrome is caused by calcified infarcts in the tegmentum of the pons and medulla oblongata occurring during fetal life or failure of the brainstem nuclei to develop. In addition to the facial weakness, most patients have drooling, dysphagia, dysarthria and bilateral paralysis of the abducens nerve causing paralysis of eye abduction.

☑ Conditions often mistaken as facial weakness include hemihypertrophy (congenital overgrowth often involving the size or length of extremities, but may involve the face) and Goldenhar syndrome (oculo-auriculo-vertebral with hypoplastic malar and maxilla on one side and sensory neural deafness) due to defect of the first two branchial arches.

☑ CANOMAD syndrome is a rare immune-mediated demyelinating polyneuropathy caused by disialosyl antibodies.

☑ Facial palsy in neonates is not apparent until crying, when the facial asymmetry becomes obvious.

☑ In Lyme disease, caused by the spirochete *Borrelia burgdorferi*, facial nerve palsy is common and it may be the initial or the only manifestation of the disease.

☑ Agenesis of depressor angularis oris muscle – also termed asymmetric facial crying or congenital unilateral lower lip palsy (CULLP) – is a congenital defect due to underdevelopment of the muscle controlling the lip. It is often mistaken as facial palsy but the lesion is permanent.

Red flags

☑ Facial seventh nerve palsy may occur during the course of acute or chronic otitis media. Myringotomy with culture of the middle-ear fluid should be carried out and parenteral antibiotics are urgently required.

☑ Beware that if there is no recovery of the Bell's palsy within a few weeks, electrophysiological examination of the facial nerve is indicated to determine the degree of neuropathy and regeneration. Neuroimaging is also indicated to exclude tumour such as neurofibroma.

☑ Note that because patients are not able to close the eye on the affected side of facial palsy, protection of the cornea with eye drops, particularly at night, is of paramount importance.

☑ An uncommon cause of facial weakness is acoustic neuroma, occurring either as a sporadic form or in association with an inherited form of neurofibromatosis type 2. Children present with hearing loss (the most common symptom in 95%), vertigo and tinnitus.

NOTES:

General physical

Excessive crying (including baby colic)

Tiredness/fatigue

Excessive weight gain

Failure to thrive and weight loss

Short stature

Excessive height

Intellectual disability (developmental delay)

EXCESSIVE CRYING (INCLUDING BABY COLIC)

The clinician overview

Although there is no agreed definition for excessive crying, it is common and normal for infants to cry up to 2 hours a day. Colic is not a diagnosis; it is simply a term that describes infants with paroxysmal excessive crying for no apparent reason, presumably of intestinal origin, during the first 3–4 months. It is defined as crying for over 3 hours a day, over 3 days a week and for over 3 weeks. It usually begins around the age of 2 weeks and significantly improves by the age of 3–4 months. Characteristically, the attack begins suddenly, is continuous, with flushed face, tense abdomen, fisted hands and drawing up of legs towards the abdomen. Crying may be considered as a baby's way of communication. As children grow older, they find different ways to communicate.

Possible diagnoses

INFANTS
Common
- Colic (evening or 3-months colic)
- Discomfort (too warm or too cold, nappy rash)
- GO reflux
- Infection (e.g. otitis media (OM))
- Milk and food allergy/intolerance

Rare
- Non-accidental injury
- Intestinal obstruction (e.g. intussusception)
- Constipation
- Teething
- Hypoxia
- Peritonitis

CHILDREN
- Pain (e.g. abdominal pain)
- Food intolerance (including milk intolerance)
- GO reflux
- Infection (e.g. OM)
- Night terror

- Non-accidental injury
- Intestinal obstruction (e.g. intussusception)
- Anxiety
- Renal stones or gallstones
- Threadworms
- Peritonitis
- Constipation

Differential diagnosis at a glance

	Pain	Food intolerance	GO reflux	Infection	Night terror
Mainly at night	Possible	No	No	No	Yes
Related to food intake	Possible	Yes	Yes	No	No
Fever present	Possible	No	No	Yes	No
Associated vomiting	Possible	Possible	Yes	Possible	No
Persisting for weeks	Possible	Yes	Yes	No	Possible

Recommended investigations

There are usually no tests needed. Occasionally, some tests may be required including the following.

***   Urine for UTI with dipsticks; discard if nitrate and leukocytes are negative.

**   FBC, CRP for infection such as appendicitis.

***   Plain X-ray of abdomen for intestinal obstruction, e.g. intussusception.

***   Abdominal ultrasound scan for suspected intestinal pathology such as intestinal obstruction.

**   pH-probe study will diagnose GO reflux (in mild cases diagnosis is made by response to therapy).

TOP TIPS

◪ Evening colic (3-months colic) used to be the most common diagnosis of infantile colic; this is being replaced by GO reflux.

◪ Colic typically is noted in the afternoon and evening (commonly 6 p.m.–10 p.m.) suggesting that events at home (e.g. mum is busy with households; child being left alone) could be the major cause.

◪ A sympathetic and supportive clinician who has time to listen to parental concerns of excessive crying is a prerequisite for a successful management.

◪ Although several over-the-counter preparations are used for colic (gripe water, Infacol, dentinox), they are scientifically not proven.

◪ Sedation or temporary hospital admission is occasionally required for babies with excessive crying. This is done if other measures fail and often for maternal indication, i.e. to give relief to an exhausted mother.

◪ Examination of an infant's abdomen is only diagnostically rewarding when the child is not in an episode of colic.

Red
flags

- The diagnosis of colic should not be made without excluding more serious disorders such as OM or intussusception.
- Beware the possibility of non-accidental injury for unexplained baby crying. Check the baby's weight for a possible FTT and the skin for any bruises.
- A child who develops severe paroxysmal abdominal pain after the age of 3 months should carefully be examined to exclude intussusception.
- Beware that the fontanel can be bulging when the baby is crying; if it remains so after cessation of crying, this sign is serious and occurs in meningitis or hydrocephalus.
- The administration of a sedative to a child with persistent crying may mask an underlying abdominal pathology; it should be the last resort.

NOTES:

TIREDNESS/FATIGUE

The clinician overview

Most childhood diseases, particularly infections, cause fatigue, which may last for many days and sometimes weeks. Chronic fatigue syndrome (CFS) is defined as an unexplained fatigue, not relieved by rest, with significant impairment of function and participation, excluding other underlying causative disorders (including psychological and psychiatric diseases) and lasting for a minimum of 6 months. The fatigue is usually debilitating, but often fluctuating in intensity, and typically exacerbated by exercise or activity. It can cause considerable morbidity and impaired emotional stability and social development. The condition is rare before the age of 10 years.

Possible diagnoses

INFANTS
Common
- Chronic respiratory diseases
- Cardiac diseases
- Drugs (e.g. antiepileptics)
- Neuromuscular diseases
- Chronic infection/inflammation

Rare
- Malnutrition/chronic anaemia
- Botulism
- Malignancy
- Obstructive sleep apnoea
- Hypokalaemia

CHILDREN

- CFS
- Post-viral fatigue
- Drugs (e.g. antihistamine, antiepileptics)
- Psychiatric illness (e.g. depression, anxiety disorder)
- Chronic infection/inflammation

- Autoimmune disease (e.g. systemic lupus erythematosus (SLE))
- Neuromuscular diseases (e.g. myasthenia)
- Obstructive sleep apnoea
- Gastrointestinal diseases (e.g. coeliac disease)
- Malnutrition/chronic anaemia (e.g. iron-deficiency anaemia)
- Endocrine disorders (e.g. Addison's, hypothyroidism)
- Occult malignancy (e.g. lymphoma, neuroblastoma)
- Fibromyalgia fibrositis

- Inflammatory bowel diseases (e.g. Crohn's disease)
- Botulism
- Hypokalaemia

Differential diagnosis at a glance

	CFS	Post-viral fatigue	Drugs	Psychiatric illness	Chronic infection/ inflammation
Preceded by a viral infection	Possible	Yes	No	No	Possible
Presence of delusions and hallucinations	No	No	No	Yes	No
Symptoms for > 6 months	Yes	No	Possible	Possible	Possible
Rest relieves fatigue	No	Possible	Yes	Possible	Yes
High ESR and CRP	No	No	No	No	Possible

Recommended investigations

***   Urine: proteinuria in renal abnormalities such as CRF and tubular acidosis.

***   FBC: Hb for chronic anaemia and infection; WBC for infection.

**   ESR/CRP: high level suggests autoimmune diseases (e.g. SLE), or chronic infection (e.g. TB).

***   U&E: deranged in renal impairment and hypokalaemia.

***   LFTs for chronic infection, jaundice, anaemia.

***   TFTs will confirm hypothyroidism (early clinical signs of hypothyroidism may be subtle).

***   CPK for evidence of muscle disease.

***   Serology for coeliac disease, toxoplasmosis, Lyme disease.

**   Autoimmune screening tests such as ANAs.

***   IgM for toxoplasmosis, Epstein–Barr virus (EBV), cytomegalovirus, HHV-6.

**   Drug levels in blood for antiepileptics and for possible illicit drugs.

**   Serological tests for Lyme disease (IgM).

***   Mantoux test for chronic infection and suspected TB.

***   Chest X-ray for possible lymphoma.

TOP TIPS

- CFS should be differentiated from post-viral fatigue; the latter is of short duration in addition to a clear history of an infection at onset with laboratory evidence of a viral infection.
- A child is best managed in CFS centres, which are led by CFS specialists. In 2004, 13 new centres in the United Kingdom were established with the aim to improve the care of CFS sufferers.
- CFS can be an extremely isolating illness. If the patient and parents wish, establishing contacts with a patient support group can be very helpful for overcoming isolation and providing contact with similar-aged patients.
- While fibromyalgia is characterised by widespread musculoskeletal pain (generalised or localised), and joint tenderness, the associated fatigue is mild in contrast to that in CFS which is prominent.
- If the history and physical examination suggest CFS, the patient and family should be told that CFS is a possibility, and why investigations are being carried out.
- Clinicians should be prepared to ask an experienced colleague for a second opinion if they, the patient or the parents have doubt about the diagnosis of CFS.
- CFS should not be made in patients with prior history of depressive or psychotic disorders such as schizophrenia.
- Clinicians should be prepared to refer patients to another health service for further investigation, symptom control or for the implementation of a multidisciplinary management plan.
- Requesting viral titres for many viruses is not recommended apart from IgM and IgG for EBV.
- Antidepressants should only be prescribed if there is severe mood disorder and after consultation with a psychiatrist.

- In myasthenia gravis, the fatigue is characteristically late in the day or after exercise; ptosis is a typical presentation.
- Beware that patients often have sleep disturbance; so a good history of the sleep pattern is essential.

NOTES:

EXCESSIVE WEIGHT GAIN

The clinician overview

Obesity is a very common and serious problem in children, with important implications for the child's health, including emotional health, and for health services. It is linked to adult obesity with the potential risk of increased mortality, cardiovascular disease, hypertension, diabetes, back pain, hyperlipidaemia, cholelithiasis and sleep apnoea. Obese children often do not eat more than their peers. Genetic factors and reduced energy output (long hours sitting in front of TV and computer) are more important causal factors. Obesity is usually the result of increases in the number of fat cells (adipocytes) occurring during gestational months and during the first year of life. Any early obesity may persist. Other causes of obesity, including hormonal and endocrine, are rare in clinical practice but often considered to be the reason by parents.

Possible diagnoses

INFANTS
Common

- Obese mother
- Infant of diabetic mother
- Post-term infants
- Oedema (cardiac or renal)
- Drugs (e.g. steroids)

CHILDREN

- Simple obesity
- Polycystic ovary syndrome (POS)
- Endocrine (e.g. Cushing's syndrome (CS), hypothyroidism)
- Genetic syndromes (e.g. Turner's and Prader–Willi syndromes)
- Drugs (e.g. steroids, pizotifen, anticonvulsants)

Rare

- Insulinoma
- Beckwith–Wiedemann syndrome (associated with hypoglycaemia)
- Cerebral gigantism (Sotos syndrome)

- Cerebral gigantism (Sotos syndrome)
- Oedema (renal or cardiac)
- Beckwith–Wiedemann syndrome
- Laurence–Moon–Biedl syndrome (polydactyly, learning disability, retinitis pigmentosa)

Differential diagnosis at a glance

	Simple obesity	POS	Endocrine	Genetic syndromes	Drugs
Tall for age	Yes	Possible	No	No	Possible
Truncal striae	Possible	Possible	Yes	No	Possible
Truncal obesity	No	No	Yes	No	No
Elevated BP	No	No	Possible	Possible	Possible
Delayed bone age	No	No	Yes	Yes	Possible

Recommended investigations

***   Urine: proteinuria in case of oedema caused by renal disease; free cortisol confirms CS.

***   TFT: will confirm or exclude hypothyroidism.

***   U&E in blood: deranged in CS.

***   Blood glucose for cases with non-insulin-dependent diabetes mellitus (NIDDM) and Beckwith–Wiedemann syndrome.

***   Calcium and parathyroid hormone for cases with hypoparathyroidism.

***   Serum cortisol levels will confirm CS.

**   Bone age in obesity normal or advanced; delayed in endocrine disorders.

**   Pelvic ultrasound scan: will confirm ovarian cysts in PCOS; the adrenals for CS.

**   CT scan or MRI for suspected cases of CS.

TOP TIPS

☑ Obesity due to syndrome or endocrine causes is rare; children are differentiated from those with simple obesity by being short, have delayed bone age and delayed onset of secondary sexual characteristics.

☑ A common reason for seeking medical help for child's obesity is parental concern whether the 'child's glands' are normal. Obesity usually has no 'glands' as an underlying cause.

☑ As body mass index (BMI) gives no indication of body fat distribution, waist circumference (midway between the tenth rib and top of the iliac crest) is a marker for central body fat accumulation and is more accurate than BMI.

☑ Much time is wasted in clinic by giving unwanted advice about food. The child with obesity is aware of that, often upset by frequently hearing that they are eating too much, and dietary restriction is notoriously unsuccessful in treating the condition.

☑ The main cause of childhood-onset obesity is not overeating, but genetic (usually confirmed by a detailed family history) and decreased energy output. The latter can be estimated indirectly by the total hours spent in front of TV and computer per day.

☑ NIDDM, elevated levels of low-density lipoprotein and low levels of high-density lipoprotein occur in association with obesity and are risk factors in cardiovascular disease and stroke.

- Beware that most pre-pubertal children with obesity are tall for their age; those with endocrine causes (hypothyroidism, CS) and with Turner's or Prader–Willi syndromes, are below average in height.
- Establish whether the excessive weight is due to a simple obesity or to rare causes. In simple obesity, fat distribution is diffuse and physical examination is otherwise normal. Truncal obesity with thin legs is merely seen in adolescents or adults with CS; in young children the fat distribution may be diffuse involving the face, trunk and cervical region (buffalo hump).
- Remember that striae are unusual before teen years; they are pink in simple obesity or during rapid growth in adolescents. In CS these marks appear early and are violaceous.
- Don't miss another uncommon but important physical sign in an obese child: when the hand is fisted it may show short fourth and fifth knuckles; a sign seen in pseudohypoparathyroidism and in girls with Turner's syndrome.
- Don't miss recording blood pressure in any child with obesity; elevated in those with CS and Turner's syndrome.

- Beware that finding of supernumerary digits with obesity raises the likelihood of Laurence–Moon–Biedl syndrome (obesity, polydactyly, retinitis pigmentosa and progressive nephropathy).

NOTES:

FAILURE TO THRIVE AND WEIGHT LOSS

The clinician overview

Although there is no agreement about a definition of failure to thrive (FTT), a child whose weight is well below the third percentile (or more accurately if the weight is below 0.4 percentile on the 9 percentile chart) or a weight loss that has crossed two percentiles should be considered as FTT. It is divided into two main categories: organic and non-organic causes. In children, in contrast to adults, psychosocial causes are far more common than organic causes. If the history and physical examination do not suggest a specific underlying organic disease in a child who fails to thrive, psychosocial causes are likely and laboratory and imaging are unlikely to provide the answer.

Possible diagnoses

INFANTS
Common
- Small for date
- Emotional deprivation
- Chronic illness
- Malnutrition
- Inborn errors of metabolism

Rare

CHILDREN

- Psychosocial (e.g. emotional deprivation)
- Eating disorder (e.g. anorexia nervosa)
- Infection (e.g. HIV, parasitic)
- Malnutrition (marasmus)
- Malabsorption (e.g. coeliac disease)

- Depression, anxiety
- Inflammatory bowel disease
- Malignancy
- Malnutrition
- Endocrine (e.g. hyperthyroidism)
- HIV infection

Differential diagnosis at a glance

	Psychosocial	Eating disorder	Infection	Malnutrition	Malabsorption
Abnormal physical findings	Possible	No	Possible	Possible	Possible
Likely affecting infants and toddlers	Yes	No	Yes	Yes	Yes
Abnormal stools	No	No	Possible	Possible	Possible
Recurrent infections	Possible	No	Yes	Yes	Possible
Fear of becoming obese	No	Yes	No	No	No

Recommended investigations

***   Urine: proteinuria in renal disease.

***   FBC: looking for anaemia prevalent in malnutrition, infection and malabsorption.

**   Inflammatory markers (CRP or ESR): elevated in infectious diseases.

***   TFTs will confirm hyperthyroidism.

***   Coeliac screening tests in blood.

TOP TIPS

☑ Chronic psychosocial or physical disorder can affect the growth and development of infants and young children. Older children can be affected psychologically by frequent hospitalisation and visiting other health facilities, thus missing normal socialisation, opportunity to learn independence and responsibility for self-care. It also causes learning difficulty.

☑ Remember that while high-quality childcare with provision of love influences favourably the child's development and thriving, poor-quality care adversely affects development and thriving.

☑ Neglect, either nutritional or emotional, is the most common cause of underweight in infancy and may account for more than 50% of cases with FTT.

☑ Community paediatricians have a central role in the care of children with chronic illness and in supporting their families. The main role of paediatricians is establishing a diagnosis and arranging referrals to sub-specialties and other medical facilities.

☑ Depressive disorder occurs in about 50% of adolescents. They may show either a decrease or increase in weight.

☑ Avoid wrong diagnosis of 'growth failure' in premature infants: when plotting growth parameters, subtract the weeks of prematurity from the postnatal age.

☑ Weight loss in adolescent girls is likely to be due to an eating disorder. Diagnosis can be difficult in the early stage. Asking about attitude toward eating and weight will suggest the diagnosis.

Red flags

- ▱ Small-for-gestational-age babies (weight < 10 percentile for gestational age) dated from the first trimester (symmetrically affecting the height and head circumference as well) often remain underweight. They should not be categorised as FTT.
- ▱ Children who were small for their gestational age often have slow weight gain during the first 1–3 years of life. They have to be differentiated from those who have gained weight and then experience weight loss. The latter should be investigated.
- ▱ Beware of children at high risk of abuse: excessive crying during infancy, physical handicap, chronic illness, with behavioural or learning difficulties.
- ▱ Neglected children returning to their parents without any medical or social intervention may face serious re-injury (in about 25%) or death (in about 5%).

NOTES:

SHORT STATURE

The clinician overview

Short stature (SS) is defined as height under 2 standard deviations below the mean or under the third percentile. The three most common causes of SS worldwide are familial, constitutional delay and malnutrition. Familial SS is seen in normal children who have short parents, normal growth rate and bone age, and enter puberty at the normal time. Their ultimate height is related to their parental height. Children with constitutional delay have a normal growth rate, but delayed onset of puberty and bone age. Because of delayed bone age, children have more time to grow, and they usually achieve a normal adult height appropriate to the family pattern. Worldwide, malnutrition is the most common cause of SS. Chronic diseases causing SS are mainly due to malnutrition.

Possible diagnoses

INFANTS
Common
- Familial SS
- Skeletal abnormalities
- Malnutrition
- Emotional deprivation

Rare

CHILDREN

- Familial SS
- Constitutional delay
- Malnutrition
- Chronic disease (e.g. inflammatory bowel disease, malabsorption)
- Chromosomal (e.g. Turner's syndrome)

- Endocrine (e.g. hypothyroidism, poorly controlled diabetes)
- Emotional deprivation
- Skeletal abnormality (achondroplasia)

Differential diagnosis at a glance

	Familial SS	Constitutional delay	Malnutrition	Chronic disease	Chromosomal
Normal growth rate of > 5 cm per year	Yes	Yes	No	Possible	No
Low ratio of weight to height	No	No	Yes	Possible	No
Normal physical examination	Yes	Yes	No	No	No
Short parents	Yes	Possible	Possible	Possible	Possible
Delayed bone age	No	Yes	Yes	Yes	No

Recommended investigations

***   FBC: to exclude anaemia (common in malnutrition).
***   Blood glucose if growth hormone (GH) deficiency is suspected.
***   TFT will confirm hypothyroidism.
**   GH check, often done by checking the IGF-1.
***   LFTs, U&E if liver or renal disease is suspected.
***   Plasma gonadotropin levels: elevated in Turner's syndrome.
***   Karyotyping in girls to exclude Turner's syndrome (Karyotype 45, X.)
***   Bone age to differentiate familial SS from constitutional delay; also useful in endocrine causes.
***   Ultrasonography of the heart, kidney and ovaries for Turner's syndrome.

TOP TIPS

- Children normally have their highest growth rate from birth to 1 year of life (23–28 cm); this decreases aged 1–3 years (7.5–13 cm) and aged 3 years to puberty (5–7 cm) but increases during puberty (8–9 cm in girls and 10–10.5 cm in boys).
- Children's growth is like tree growth; they grow faster in spring and summer, therefore growth velocity should be measured for 1 year.
- Measuring the height of both parents is essential in evaluating a child with SS. It helps diagnose familial SS and predict the ultimate height of the children.
- The term SS is often confused with growth failure. SS is defined as height under the third percentile with normal annual growth rate, while growth failure is defined as a growth rate of < 5 cm per year.
- Parents of children with SS often seek medical services because of possible 'endocrine' causes; endocrine diseases are rare and no more than 5% of causes.
- In GH deficiency, the weight to height ratio is increased on the percentile chart, while it is decreased in chronic disease (inflammatory bowel disease).

■ When evaluating children with SS, it is more important how their growth rate has been rather than where the percentile is on the chart.

Red flags

■ Remember that the vast majority of short children do not have GH deficiency, but because the deficiency is potentially treatable, it must be considered carefully and excluded.
■ GH is a major counter-regulatory hormone to insulin; therefore, children with GH deficiency may present with hypoglycaemia, particularly during fasting or mild illness.
■ Always consider Turner's syndrome when pubertal delay is combined with SS. Physical signs may be subtle, and they may achieve menstrual periods as well as breast development in 10%–20%.
■ A search for an organic cause of SS should be sought if there are symptoms such as weight loss, diarrhoea, poor appetite, headaches.

NOTES:

EXCESSIVE HEIGHT

The clinician overview

Growth is influenced by many factors such as hereditary, genetic, illness, nutritional, medication, hormonal and psychological influences. As a general rule, a child's potential height ranges between the averages of the parents height. Tall parents usually have tall children. Hereditary and genetic factors are by far responsible for excessive height. Although growth hormone (GH) is known to be responsible for gigantism and acromegaly, other conditions associated with an excessive GH-secretion and possible gigantism include McCune–Albright syndrome (incidence of gigantism 15%–20%), neurofibromatosis type 1, familial somatotropinoma (autosomal dominant) and multiple endocrine neoplasia with multiple cancer (autosomal dominant).

Possible diagnoses

INFANTS
Common
- Hereditary/genetic
- Hyperinsulinism
- Large-of-date babies
- Infant of diabetic mother
- Sotos syndrome

Rare

CHILDREN

- Hereditary/genetic
- Obesity
- Klinefelter's syndrome (chromosome: 47, XXY)
- Pituitary gigantism
- Marfan's syndrome

- Sotos syndrome
- Precocious puberty (such as McCune–Albright syndrome)
- Beckwith–Wiedemann syndrome (BWS)
- Homocystinuria
- Hypogonadism

Differential diagnosis at a glance

	Hereditary/genetic	Obesity	Klinefelter's syndrome	Pituitary gigantism	Marfan's syndrome
Very tall	Possible	No	No	Possible	Possible
Tall parents	Yes	Possible	Possible	Possible	Possible
Associated with intellectual deficit	No	No	Yes	No	No
Diagnosis is likely made on examination	Yes	Yes	Possible	No	Yes
BMI > 30%	Possible	Yes	Possible	Possible	Possible

Recommended investigations

*** Urine for homocystine: increased in homocystinuria but cystine is low or absent in blood.

*** Insulin-growth factor 1 and GH in blood: elevated in pituitary gigantism and acromegaly.

** Plasma levels of FSH, LH for Klinefelter's syndrome.

*** Karyotyping for suspected cases of Klinefelter's syndrome (will show 47 chromosomes XXY).

*** Skeletal X-ray for a child with precocious puberty (e.g. McCune–Albright syndrome).

*** Echocardiography for Marfan's syndrome to exclude aneurysm.

*** Cranial MRI for suspected pituitary tall stature to exclude adenoma.

TOP TIPS

◪ Although there is no definition of excessive height, children who are above the 99.6 percentile for age and sex on the 9-percentile chart are considered as such.

◪ Remember that over 50% of obese children have a height in the 70th–99th percentile.

◪ Beware that girls are more likely than boys to report concern to their general practitioners about their height at an early age. Society perceives tall and slender girls as beautiful but excessive height as less acceptable than in boys.

◪ Although tall parents usually have tall children, remember that a tall father may be tall for another underlying cause, such as Marfan's syndrome.

◪ One important cause of tall stature is precocious puberty. The skin should be examined for café-au-lait maculae to exclude McCune–Albright syndrome, which is also associated with bone fibrous dysplasia.

Red flags

- Child's length or height must be measured accurately. In children younger than 24 months, recumbent length and standing height are not the same; the former being significantly greater. Measurement with tape is inaccurate.
- Beware that children with excessive height are at risk of developing orthopaedic problems such as kyphosis and scoliosis, and psychiatric problems such as anxiety, depression and behaviour disorders.
- Beware that children with Klinefelter's syndrome often present with complaints other than height, e.g. gynaecomastia, behaviour problems such as aggressiveness, excessive shyness and antisocial acts such as fire-setting and crimes.
- Beware that children with Marfan's syndrome are at risk of early death because of progressive aortic dilatation. Arachnodactyly and lens dislocation are important clues that need to be differentiated from patients with homocystinuria. Referral to an ophthalmologist is important.
- Overgrowth syndromes are a group of children characterised by excessive somatic growth. BWS is the most well known of these syndromes. They are predisposed to cancers such as nephroblastoma and adrenocortical carcinoma.

NOTES:

INTELLECTUAL DISABILITY (DEVELOPMENTAL DELAY)

The clinician overview

Intellectual disability (ID) is characterised by a significantly below average intellectual function, causing limitation in areas of normal activities such as communication, self-care and social adaptation. The condition is common affecting about 3% of the population, of which over 90% are categorised as mild and about 5% as severe or profound. Most children with mild disability are identified in the preschool period because of inability to communicate, inability to take care of oneself (including decision-making) and deficiency in participating in social and school activities. Traditionally, ID has been grouped as prenatal (e.g. chromosomal, genetic disorder, toxins or infection during pregnancy), natal (e.g. prematurity, hypoxic-ischaemic encephalopathy, infection) and postnatal causes (e.g. head injury, autism, and infection).

Possible diagnoses

INFANTS
Common
- ▨ Extreme prematurity
- ▨ Intracranial haemorrhage
- ▨ Infection (e.g. TORCH, meningitis)
- ▨ Metabolic (e.g. hypoglycaemia)
- ▨ HIE

Rare
- ▨ Inborn errors of metabolism
- ▨ Primary microcephaly
- ▨ Congenital central nervous system malformation
- ▨ Seizures (e.g. infantile spasm)
- ▨ Fetal alcohol syndrome
- ▨ Child abuse (physical, neglect)

CHILDREN
- ▨ Chromosomal (trisomy-21, fragile X syndrome)
- ▨ Idiopathic (no cause is identified)
- ▨ Head injury
- ▨ Autism (classical autism)
- ▨ Infection (meningitis, encephalitis)

- ▨ Genetic syndrome
- ▨ Inborn errors of metabolism
- ▨ Neurocutaneous syndrome (e.g. tuberous sclerosis)
- ▨ Child abuse
- ▨ Metabolic (hypoglycaemia, hypernatraemia

187

☑ Toxins (e.g. lead)
☑ Malnutrition

Differential diagnosis at a glance

	Chromosomal	Idiopathic	Head injury	Autism	Infection
Often identified at birth	Possible	No	No	No	Possible
Severe ID	Possible	Possible	Possible	Possible	Possible
Regression after normal development	No	No	Possible	Yes	Possible
Acute onset	No	No	Yes	No	Yes
Associated psychomotor delay	Yes	Possible	Possible	Yes	Possible

Recommended investigations

**   Urine for mucopolysaccharides; reducing substance for e.g. galactosaemia.
***   Karyotyping including with fragile X analysis.
***   Metabolic screen: blood glucose, U&E, organic acids, aminoacids, ammonia, lactate, pyruvate.
**   Serum uric acid for any boy with self-mutilation.
**   Plasma lead, copper and ceruloplasmin for Wilson's disease.
**   Viral titres for congenital infections.
**   WBC lysosomal enzyme or skin biopsy for neuro-regression, optic atrophy.
***   EEG for suspected seizure disorders.
***   Cranial MRI for focal seizures, neurocutaneous syndrome.

TOP TIPS

☑ When evaluating premature children younger than 24 months, correction for gestational age should be considered. A child at a chronological age of 12 months who was born 3 months prematurely is 9 months corrected.
☑ Mild degree of ID may not manifest until toddler age or after school entry, and is usually present with delayed speech and language development.
☑ Remember that while poor-quality childcare at home can adversely affect developmental outcome, high-quality childcare may result in improving it.
☑ In particular neglect (e.g. isolation, bullying), child abuse is recognised to cause ID. Neglect is three times more common than physical abuse and tends to occur over a long period of time.

- The long-used classification of ID based on IQ (mild: 55–69; moderate: 40–54; < 40: severe) is no longer used. In 1992 a new classification of ID was proposed, which was based on the amount of support and supervision that the individual needs: intermittent, limited, extensive and pervasive.
- The long-used term 'mental retardation' should not be used any more; there is undesirable stigma associated with this term. Intellectual disability, developmental delay or learning difficulty are far more appropriate and acceptable terms.

- The first step in evaluation of a child suspected of ID: is the hearing and vision normal? These could cause symptoms wrongly perceived as ID.
- Beware of the difference between a child who has always shown developmental delay and one who developed normally and then lost motor or cognitive skill. The latter needs an urgent evaluation as such regression could indicate a neurodegenerative disease, metabolic disorder, autism or seizure (such as infantile spasm).
- Remember that fragile X syndrome is seen in 1 in 2600 males and 1 in 4200 females; a very common sign (identified in 80%–90%) is macroorchidism (defined as a testis size of > 4 mL or > 2 times normal) which should not be missed on examination.

NOTES:

Genital

Penile swelling

Scrotal/testicular swelling and pain

Groin swelling

Vaginal discharge

Rectal prolapse

Delayed puberty

Precocious puberty

PENILE SWELLING

The clinician overview

Swelling of the penis, often with inflammation and pain, may occur in association with nappy rash or forceful attempt to retract the foreskin. Other common causes are balanitis (inflammation of the glans) and posthitis (inflammation of the prepuce). Balano-posthitis refers to inflammation of both sites. Priapism, a non-erotic, persistent unwanted erection, is a relatively frequent complication in children with sickle-cell anaemia (SCA). Trauma is another important cause of priapism, which may be high-flow due to an arterio-venous shunt or low-flow when there is obstruction to the venous outflow. The oedema of nephrotic syndrome (NS) or Henöch–Schönlein purpura (HSP) accumulates in dependent sites and often causes penile swelling. It is easy to differentiate balanitis from oedema: the later lacks redness and other inflammatory signs. Practically all cases of penile swelling require immediate medical attention.

Possible diagnoses

INFANTS
Common
- ▨ Trauma (birth injury, e.g. breech delivery)
- ▨ Balanitis
- ▨ Congenital adrenal hyperplasia
- ▨ Associated with nappy rash
- ▨ Penile oedema (idiopathic, generalised oedema)

Rare
- ▨ Congenital NS
- ▨ Paraphimosis
- ▨ Congenital lymphoedema

CHILDREN
- ▨ Balanitis
- ▨ Trauma
- ▨ Paraphimosis
- ▨ Priapism
- ▨ Penile oedema (e.g. NS, HSP)

- ▨ Drugs (cocaine, serotonin reuptake inhibitors)
- ▨ Penile torsion
- ▨ Para-urethral cyst
- ▨ Congenital or post-infectious lymphoedema
- ▨ Tumour (including carcinoma)
- ▨ Megalourethra (with abnormal development of the corpus spongiosum)
- ▨ Epidermal inclusion cyst

☑ Condom-induced allergy (latex allergy)

Differential diagnosis at a glance

	Balanitis	Trauma	Paraphimosis	Priapism	Penile oedema
Inflammatory changes (e.g. redness)	Yes	Possible	No	No	No
Associated systemic disease	No	Possible	No	Yes	Possible
Urethral discharge	Possible	Possible	No	No	No
Engorgement of glans only	Possible	No	Yes	No	No
Tenderness	Yes	Yes	Yes	Yes	No

Recommended investigations

***   Urine to confirm proteinuria in case of NS.

***   Hormonal tests to exclude congenital adrenal hyperplasia (CAH) such as plasma 17-hydroxyprogesterone.

***   Hb, Hb-electrophoresis and peripheral blood film for any non-traumatic priapism.

***   Plasma albumin, cholesterol and triglycerides for cases of NS.

***   Gram-stained smear and culture in case of urethral discharge.

TOP TIPS

☑ Remember that the foreskin is normally non-retractile and attached to the glans in most neonates. It becomes retractile in about 40% of children aged 1 year, 90% aged 4 years and 99% aged 15 years.

☑ Balanitis, the most common cause of penile inflammation, may result from allergy, seborrhoeic dermatitis, insect bites or from any erosion of the skin allowing bacteria (usually staphylococci) to invade. STD should be considered in sexually active adolescents.

☑ Priapism in SCA results from pooling of blood in the corpora cavernosa causing obstruction to the venous outflow. It usually lasts more than 4 hours.

☑ A rare condition of penile swelling is penile torsion, which is a rotation of the penis, usually in anticlockwise fashion.

☑ Immediate management of children with priapism includes ice packs, bed rest, emptying the bladder, oral or IV hydration, analgesics. Morphine may be required.

☑ Note that the oedema in NS is initially subtle, appearing around the eyes and in the lower legs, but the penile swelling is more recognisable and may be the first initial sign of the disease.

Red flags

☑ Although SCA is the most common and well-known cause of priapism, penile neoplasms, leukaemia (particularly chronic granulocytic leukaemia), cocaine abuse and scorpion bite are other, rarer, causes.

☑ Attempt to forcefully retract the foreskin (e.g. for cleansing) is dangerous; this can lead to balanitis or paraphimosis.

☑ An enlarged penis at birth may be the only clinical manifestation of CAH as some degrees of masculinisation is almost always present at birth. In girls, enlargement of the clitoris and labial fusion dominate the clinical features of CAH at birth.

☑ Beware that cases of paraphimosis (a retracted foreskin behind the corona glandis that cannot be returned) require immediate attention if ischaemia of the glans is to be prevented. Firm manual compression, with local anaesthetic cream and gauze, will usually reduce the constriction.

☑ Parents of children with SCA should be informed of priapism as a possible complication of SCA and told to seek immediate medical assistance if it occurs.

☑ Priapism requires immediate medical assistance as it can lead to ischaemia, erectile dysfunction and impotence in the future.

NOTES:

SCROTAL/TESTICULAR SWELLING AND PAIN

The clinician overview

Scrotal swelling is very common in children and may be acute or chronic, painful or painless. The two most common painless causes are hydrocele and inguinal hernia. Hydrocele is caused by drainage of peritoneal fluid through a narrow patent processus vaginalis, while inguinal hernia is due to a wide patent processus vaginalis that allows omentum or bowel to pass into the scrotum. Inguinal hernia is frequently associated with undescended testes, prematurity and connective tissue diseases such as Marfan's syndrome. The four most common painful causes of testicular swelling are testicular torsion, torsion of testicular appendage, incarcerated inguinal hernia and epididymitis/orchitis. These cases need urgent evaluation and surgical consultation.

Possible diagnoses

INFANTS
Common
- Hydrocele
- Inguinal hernia
- Birth trauma affecting the genitalia
- Epididymitis/orchitis
- Drainage from ascites

Rare
- Testicular torsion
- Generalised oedema (e.g. nephrotic syndrome (NS))
- Testicular tumour (e.g. hamartoma)
- Generalised oedema (NS)
- Torsion of the spermatic cord
- Varicocele
- Vasculitis (Henöch–Schönlein purpura, Kawasaki's disease)

CHILDREN

- Hydrocele
- Inguinal hernia
- Testicular torsion
- Epididymitis/orchitis
- Torsion of testicular appendix

- Testicular tumour (germ- and non-germ-cell tumour)
- Trauma (scrotal haematoma)
- Idiopathic scrotal oedema (ISO)

Differential diagnosis at a glance

	Hydrocele	Inguinal hernia	Testicular torsion	Epididymitis/ orchitis	Torsion of testicular appendix
Pain/tender	No	No	Yes	Yes	Yes
Transilluminates	Yes	Yes	No	No	No
Common under 10 years	Yes	Yes	No	Possible	Yes
Fever/vomiting	No	No	Yes	Possible	Possible
Acute onset	No	No	Yes	Yes	Yes

Recommended investigations

***   Urinalysis may suggest associated urinary tract infection in epididymitis, proteinuria for NS.

***   Gram-stained smear and culture from any urethral discharge to exclude STD.

***   Plasma albumin, U&E and cholesterol for NS.

**   Plasma α-fetoprotein for any malignant testicular tumour (usually elevated).

**   Ultrasonography may be a help in some cases whether testis is present or merely hydrocele.

**   Colour Doppler ultrasonography assesses the testicular morphology and testicular blood flow.

**   CT or MRI scan may delineate some testicular tumour pre-operatively.

TOP TIPS

- In a mobile child with hydrocele, the size characteristically increases during daytime and decreases over nighttime.
- Torsion of testicular appendix can be differentiated from testicular torsion by the blue dot sign, which is a necrotic appendage after undergoing torsion.
- Remember that epididymitis is the most common cause of scrotal swelling in sexually active young adolescents. This is an ascending infection from the urethra.
- ISO, usually caused by allergy, may mimic torsion. The scrotum is swollen and red in ISO, there are no symptoms and testis characteristically feels normal and not tender. ISO often extends to the groin and perineum. Parents can be reassured that the swelling will disappear within a few days (without treatment), leaving some purpuric discolouration.
- Varicocele occurs in about 5% of all adolescent boys and is a common cause of subfertility.

Red flags

- Beware that torsion of testis in neonates may be asymptomatic except for red scrotal swelling.
- In suspected cases of testicular torsion, clinicians should not request any imaging or test before surgical consultation. The diagnosis is clinical and imaging is usually unnecessary. Surgical exploration is urgent.
- Abrupt onset of painful scrotal swelling is usually caused by incarcerated hernia or testicular torsion. The onset of pain in torsion of testicular appendix is usually gradual.
- Epididymitis/orchitis may mimic testicular torsion; the inflammation, however, is commonly secondary to viral infection (e.g. mumps) or STD. In addition, the pain is more gradual in epididymitis/orchitis, nausea and vomiting is uncommon, and it is often associated with fever, dysuria and pyuria.
- Torsion of testicular appendix usually occurs in young children under 10 years of age while testicular torsion occurs in those older than 10 years of age. If diagnosis is uncertain, scrotal exploration is required in both.

NOTES:

GROIN SWELLING

The clinician overview

The mother usually notices swelling of the groin in infants and young children while giving the child a bath. Lymphadenopathy and inguinal hernia (IH) are the two most common causes. An important finding in this area is spermatic cord hydrocele, which is a fluid collection along the spermatic cord; it results from abnormal closure of the processus vaginalis and is separated from the testis and epididymis. It has two types: an encysted hydrocele, which does not communicate with the peritoneum, and a communicating hydrocele, where the fluid collection communicates with the peritoneum. Lymphadenopathy is mostly caused by local inflammation such as nappy rash.

Possible diagnoses

INFANTS
Common
- [x] IH
- [x] Lymphadenopathy (from nappy rash)
- [x] Hydrocele of spermatic cord
- [x] Undescended testis
- [x] Testicular feminisation

Rare

CHILDREN
- [x] IH
- [x] Infectious lymphadenopathy
- [x] Hydrocele of spermatic cord
- [x] Undescended testis (true undescended)
- [x] Femoral hernia

- [x] Cancerous lymphadenopathy
- [x] Testicular feminisation

Differential diagnosis at a glance

	IH	Infectious lymphadenopathy	Hydrocele of spermatic cord	Undescended testis	Femoral hernia
Reducible	Yes	No	No	No	Yes
Transilluminates	Yes	No	Yes	No	Yes
Bilateral	Possible	Possible	Possible	Possible	No
May change its size daily	Yes	No	Possible	No	Possible
Empty scrotum on same side	No	No	No	Yes	No

Recommended investigations

Diagnosis of groin swelling is clinical and investigations are usually not required.

*** FBC and CRP are required if the lymphadenitis is suspected to be caused by bacteria or leukaemia.

*** Ultrasound scan is useful in differentiating solid mass (lymph node from hydrocele or hernia).

*** Further tests (such as biopsy) may be required if the lymphadenopathy suggests malignancy.

TOP TIPS

- Children with cystic fibrosis, undescended testes, connective tissue diseases and prematurity (up to 30% of very low birth infants) have a very high incidence of IH.
- Transillumination simply demonstrates the presence of fluid and, of itself, is rarely diagnostic.
- It is important to differentiate between true undescended and retractile (yo-yo) testis. The scrotum in the latter is well developed while hypoplastic in true undescended, and the testis can be manipulated down into the normal scrotal position.
- As undescended testis and IH commonly coexist (both due to patent processus vaginalis) an orchidopexy is usually carried out at the time of hernia repair.
- Remember that although a child has around 600 lymph nodes, only the minority of them can be palpated mainly in the neck, sub-mandibular, axillary and inguinal regions. Generalised lymphadenopathy indicates the involvement of at least two of these sites.
- Following a repair of IH, a contralateral hernia develops in about 30%–40%. The risk rises to 50% if the repair of unilateral hernia is performed within the first year of life.

Red flags

- The risk of incarceration from an IH is high during the first 6 months of life; therefore, surgical consultation should be sought for any neonate found to have IH before leaving the hospital.
- In adults, it is a common practice to insert the index finger into the inguinal canal to feel for an impulse while the patient is asked to strain or cough. Do not do that in children; the procedure is painful and rarely yields any useful information.
- Unlike umbilical hernias, IH in children is potentially serious. They require repair as soon as possible. They do not disappear spontaneously. Referral to surgeons is urgent if the child is younger than 6 months of age.
- An IH that cannot be reduced by manipulation (this occurs in about 5%–10%) is often due to a narrow processus vaginalis and not necessarily due to incarceration. This latter complication is associated with marked tenderness, a firm mass and a child who inconsolably cries.
- IH in girls is far less common than in boys. A lump in the inguinal area may contain an ovary or, rarely, a testicle. The latter suggests testicular feminisation, which is confirmed by chromosomal analysis showing '46, XY'. There is a high incidence of later malignancy in the gonads; it is therefore routine practice to remove them once the diagnosis is established.
- Beware that stony hard lymph nodes usually suggest malignancy, often metastasis.

NOTES:

VAGINAL DISCHARGE

The clinician overview

Vaginal discharge (VD) is the most common gynaecological problem in children and adolescents. Physiologically, it occurs in neonate girls who often experience vaginal discharge (pseudo-menstruation) as a result of withdrawal of the maternal oestrogen hormone. A rise of oestrogen at the onset of puberty causes another physiological discharge (leukorrhoea). Pathological conditions of VD include non-specific VD (occurring in up to 70% of girls), which is caused by poor perineal hygiene, tendency of the labia minora to open on squatting, and close proximity of the anal orifice to the vagina allowing transfer of faecal bacteria to the vagina. Other contributory factors include the use of systemic antibiotics and steroids, wearing tight-fitting clothes such as tights, and the use of irritants such as detergents and bubble bath. Children with VD present with pruritus, frequent urination, dysuria, enuresis, sleep disturbance or erythema of the vulva. Sexual abuse is a serious problem and a high index of suspicion is required to make the diagnosis.

Possible diagnoses

INFANTS
Common
- Physiological
- Candida infection
- Seborrhoeic dermatitis
- Atopic dermatitis
- Vulvar psoriasis

Rare
- Urethral prolapse

CHILDREN

- Physiological
- Non-specific vulvovaginitis
- STD
- Foreign body (FB)
- Child abuse

- Candida infection
- Contact and allergic dermatitis
- Threadworms
- Trauma
- Lichen sclerosus
- Lichen planus
- Scabies
- Urethral prolapse
- Rhabdomyosarcoma

☑ Shigellosis

Differential diagnosis at a glance

	Physiological	Non-specific vulvovaginitis	STD	FB	Child abuse
Foul odour	No	Possible	Yes	Yes	Possible
Associated erythema	No	Yes	Yes	Yes	Possible
Contains bacteria	No	Possible	Yes	Possible	Possible
Tear/laceration	No	No	Possible	No	Yes
Likely post-pubertal	Possible	No	Yes	Possible	No

Recommended investigations

***   Urine sample for dipsticks and, if abnormal, culture.

***   Swab from the discharge for Gram stain and culture, and for candida.

**   Adhesive tape test to detect worm ova.

**   Imaging occasionally is required, e.g. for suspected FB or tumour.

TOP TIPS

☑ The non-specific discharge is typically brown or green, has a fetid odour and may be associated with bacterial infection secondary to faecal contamination.

☑ Threadworm infection typically causes recurrent vulvovaginitis and manifests as nocturnal scratching due to female worms depositing eggs on the perineum.

☑ Discharge caused by candida infection is rare before puberty but may occur in infancy. Risk factors in later age include systemic use of antibiotics and steroids.

☑ Child abuse refers to the use of children in sexual activities (including fondling, masturbation, penetration) that they do not understand or give consent to.

☑ Remember that most perpetrators of child abuse are family members, close relatives or friends who typically began relating to the child during non-sexual activities to gain the child's trust.

☑ Lichen sclerosus is characterised by a sharply demarcated area of hypopigmentation around the vulva and the perianal area. It is associated with intense itching and bleeds easily with normal toilet activities such as genital wiping.

Red flags

- Note that the majority of cases of physical examination on children suspected of child abuse do not yield abnormal findings. This does not exclude child abuse.
- Be aware that the physiological discharge and bleeding in neonate girls is usually creamy white and subsides when the child is 2 weeks of age. Any discharge or bleeding after 2–3 weeks warrants investigation.
- FB should always be considered when the discharge has a foul odour. Common objects include clumped toilet tissue or small parts of toys. Examination under general anaesthesia may be indicated.
- Beware that children suffering from child abuse may present with symptoms not related directly to their genitalia. These include sleep disturbance, non-specific behaviour changes, phobias, anorexia, poor school performance and social withdrawal. Later on, victims often present with post-traumatic stress disorder.
- The interview of the child suspected of being sexually abused is the most valuable component of medical evaluation, using the child's words for body parts, drawings and age-appropriate questions. Clinicians should not conduct the interview unless they have skill and experience in this area.
- Urinary tract infection (UTI) is very common in association with VD. Unless the UTI and/or threadworms are treated, treatment for VD is inadequate and VD will recur.

NOTES:

RECTAL PROLAPSE

The clinician overview

Rectal prolapse (RP) refers to a protrusion of the rectal mucosa through the anus; when the protrusion includes the rectal wall, it is termed procidentia. Most cases occur during the first few years of life, particularly during infancy, but rarely in older children. It is usually noted after defecation and is reduced either spontaneously or with the help of the child's own or parent's finger. It rarely becomes chronic; if it does, complications such as ulceration, bleeding and inflammation (proctitis) are likely consequences. One of the most important causes of RP is cystic fibrosis (CF) and RP may be the first manifestation of the disease.

Possible diagnoses

INFANTS
Common

- CF
- Chronic diarrhoea (coeliac, infective GE)
- Malnutrition
- Idiopathic
- Parasitic infection

Rare

- CTDs
- Chronic cough
- Repair of imperforate anus
- Meningomyelocele

CHILDREN

- Idiopathic
- CF
- Chronic constipation
- Chronic diarrhoea (e.g. ulcerative colitis)
- Connective tissue diseases (CTDs) (e.g. Ehlers–Danlos syndrome)

- Intestinal parasites
- Malnutrition
- Chronic cough (e.g. pertussis)
- Hirschsprung's disease
- Repair of imperforate anus
- Meningomyelocele

Differential diagnosis at a glance

	Idiopathic	CF	Chronic constipation	Chronic diarrhoea	CTDs
Other organ involvement	No	Yes	Possible	Possible	Yes
Underweight	No	Possible	No	Yes	Possible
Cause clear from the history	No	Yes	Yes	Yes	Possible
Readily responds to treatment	Possible	Possible	Yes	Possible	Possible
Likely in infancy	Possible	Yes	Possible	Possible	Possible

Recommended investigations

***   Screening tests in blood for coeliac disease (CD).
***   Stool for culture, search for parasites.
**   Chest X-ray and nasopharyngeal swab in cases with chronic cough.
***   Sweat test for CF.
***   Rectoscopy/sigmoidoscopy with biopsy for cases with chronic diarrhoea (e.g. ulcerative colitis).

TOP TIPS

▱ RP is more common in tropical and developing countries, due to high prevalence of diarrhoea, malnutrition and parasitic infestation.

▱ Once the cause of the RP is established, the best advice is to avoid panic; the prolapse is likely to recur, so children or parents have to learn how to reduce it.

▱ Chronic constipation is a common cause of RP; fibre-rich diet and stool softener should help.

▱ Remember that CF is one of the most common causes of RP; about 20% of CF patients have RP.

▱ Parents have to be taught how to reduce the prolapse at home and told to seek medical assistance if this is not achieved.

▱ A sweat test is indicated in all children with RP who present without a known underlying cause.

▱ In contrast to adults, incidence and recurrence of RP decreases as children grow older, and conservative management is usually successful and indicated.

- Prolonged sitting on a child's potty and straining predisposes for RP; these should be avoided.
- RP is usually painless or associated with mild discomfort; pain suggests complications such as ulceration, ischaemia or proctitis.
- RP has to be differentiated from rarer causes of prolapse resembling RP: prolapsed intussusception, haemorrhoids and prolapsed polyp. The latter appears as a dark, plum-coloured mass in contrast to the lighter pink mucosa appearance of the RP.

NOTES:

DELAYED PUBERTY

The clinician overview

Normally, menarche occurs at the median age of 13 years and usually starts 2–3 years after the start of breast enlargement (thelarche). Penile and scrotal enlargement usually occurs 1 year after the testicular enlargement. Delayed puberty (DP) is arbitrarily defined as delay of pubertal changes beyond 14 years in girls and 16 years in boys. The definition also includes those children who do not complete their puberty within 5 years from its start. The cause of DP in the vast majority of boys and in most girls is constitutional. DP is usually associated with delayed growth and velocity for chronological age. The exceptions to that are boys with Klinefelter's syndrome (47, XXY, gonadal dysgenesis), who are tall with long arms and legs, having normal adrenarche but small testes.

Possible diagnoses

INFANTS

Common

CHILDREN

- Constitutional
- Chronic diseases (malnutrition, Crohn's disease, coeliac disease, cystic fibrosis, anorexia nervosa)
- Intensive physical exercise
- Chromosomal (Turner's, Noonan's and Klinefelter's syndromes)
- Polycystic ovarian syndrome (POS)

Rare

- Central nervous system tumour (craniopharyngioma, meningioma)
- Prader–Willi syndrome
- Hyperprolactinaemia
- Infection (mumps)
- Irradiation of the gonads, chemotherapy
- Following bone marrow transplantation
- Testicular feminisation syndrome
- Chronic psychiatric disorders

Differential diagnosis at a glance

	Constitutional	Chronic diseases	Intensive physical exercise	Chromosomal	POS
Otherwise healthy	Yes	No	Yes	No	No
Short	Possible	Yes	Possible	Possible	Possible
+ family history	Yes	Possible	No	Possible	No
Underweight	Possible	Yes	Yes	No	No
Delayed bone age	Yes	Yes	Possible	Possible	No

Recommended investigations

*** FBC: Hb, ferritin, CRP (anaemia with high CRP suggests Crohn's disease).

*** Screening blood tests for coeliac disease.

*** Hormonal assay: levels of FSH/LH, gonadotropins-releasing hormone, oestrogen, testosterone, prolactin, growth hormone.

*** 17-hydroxyprogesterone and DHEAS assay for congenital adrenal hyperplasia.

*** TFTs for suspected thyroid disorders.

*** Karyotyping for suspected cases of Turner's syndrome (45, X) and Klinefelter's syndrome (XXY).

*** Wrist X-ray for bone age.

*** Pelvic ultrasound scan to detect ovarian cysts or tumour or testicular tumour.

*** Radiological investigation for suspected case of Crohn's disease.

TOP TIPS

◪ With detailed history and examination, including growth measurement, diagnosis can be established in most cases.

◪ While the principal cause of DP in boys is constitutional, girls have more frequent pathological causes, e.g. anorexia nervosa, chronic diseases, intensive exercise or chromosomal abnormalities.

◪ Puberty can easily be assessed by bone age (wrist X-ray): if bone age is within 1 year of chronological age, puberty has either not or only just started; bone age exceeding chronological age by more than one year indicates the child is in puberty.

◪ Hormonal treatment is often indicated in boys in constitutional DP (with oxandrolone aged 11.5 years and testosterone aged over 13.5 years) and in girls (with ethinylestradiol or oestrogens) if the DP and/or growth are causing distress or school underperformance.

◪ Remember this: use Tanner growth chart for pubertal stages and never forget to obtain the height of the parents and siblings when a child presents with DP.

- ◩ Once constitutional DP is established, children can be reassured that DP is inherited and physiological, and they will achieve later normal puberty.
- ◩ Remember that girls with Turner's syndrome achieve normal adrenarche and axillary hair at appropriate age. They do not develop menstruation.
- ◩ In girls with DP and short stature, Turner's syndrome should be excluded. Pelvic ultrasound scan and chromosomal analysis should be carried out. Complete androgen insensitivity syndrome should also be considered.

Red
flags

- ◩ The diagnosis of constitutional DP should not be made before excluding pathological conditions. This is the principal aim when evaluating a child with DP.
- ◩ Beware occult chronic diseases causing DP, e.g. Crohn's and coeliac disease. Poor growth is the most important clue.
- ◩ All girls with an inguinal hernia should undergo a pelvic ultrasound examination before the operation to exclude testicular feminisation (currently termed androgen insensitivity syndrome).
- ◩ In girls with otherwise normal sexual maturation but delayed menarche and galactorrhoea, prolactinoma is likely. Urgent prolactin level and MRI of the brain should be considered.

NOTES:

PRECOCIOUS PUBERTY

The clinician overview

Normal sexual development begins in girls with breast development, followed by the appearance of pubic hair (sometimes simultaneously with breast development), axillary hair, onset of menstruation, acne and adult body odour. In boys, it begins with testicular enlargement followed by enlargement of the penis, the appearance of pubic hair, deepening of the voice, acne and adult body odour. Precocious puberty (PP) is defined as puberty occurring at an unusual age, i.e. before the age of 8 years in girls or before 9 years in boys. Puberty nowadays starts earlier than in previous generations. Puberty depends on gonadotropins-releasing hormone (GnRH) through luteinising hormone release and sex hormone production. The causes of PP are best divided into central (idiopathic or with identifiable causes), adrenal and gonadal causes. In more than 90% of girls and 50% of boys, the cause of PP is idiopathic, i.e. no identifiable cause. Even in idiopathic instances, PP is often a cause of adverse effects on social behaviour and psychological development. In addition, the early growth spurt can initially cause rapid bone maturation but the linear growth ceases early, ultimately resulting in short stature. The appearance of secondary sexual characteristics should not be confused with true PP.

Possible diagnoses

INFANTS
Common
- Central nervous system injury (birth injury, hydrocephalus)
- Adrenal (e.g. congenital adrenal hyperplasia (CAH))
- Ovarian (e.g. McCune–Albright syndrome)
- Iatrogenic (external sex hormones)
- PPP (e.g. premature thelarche)

Rare

CHILDREN
- Partial PP (e.g. premature thelarche)
- Central idiopathic
- Central with identifiable causes (e.g. hamartoma)
- Gonads (ovarian cysts, McCune–Albright syndrome)
- Adrenal (e.g. congenital adrenal hyperplasia, tumour)

- Iatrogenic (external sources of sex hormones)
- Irradiation of the brain
- Familial PP in males
- Teratoma (e.g. in the mediastinum)

Differential diagnosis at a glance

	PPP	Central idiopathic	Central with identifiable causes	Gonads	Adrenal
Small testicle	Yes	No	No	Yes	Yes
Suppressed gonadotropins	No	No	No	Yes	Yes
Advanced growth and bone age	No	Yes	Yes	Yes	Yes
Non-progressive precocity	Yes	Possible	Possible	Possible	Possible
Girls > boys	Yes	Yes	Yes	Yes	No

Recommended investigations

***   Hormonal assay of GnRH, luteinising hormone (LH), follicle-stimulating hormone (FSH) and sex hormones.

***   GnRH stimulation test (in central PP, the LH and FSH levels are increased).

***   Serum level of I7-hydroxyprogesterone, DHEAS, cortisol and aldosterone in cases of CAH.

***   Wrist X-ray to assess bone maturation.

***   Pelvic ultrasound scan and adrenal visualisation for CAH.

***   CT scan or MRI of the head for all cases suspected of central causes of PP.

**   Skeletal survey for bony fibrous dysplasia for a child with PP and hyperpigmented spots.

TOP TIPS

☑ Puberty can easily be assessed by bone age (wrist X-ray): if bone age is within 1 year of chronological age, puberty either has not or just started; bone age exceeding chronological age by more than one year indicates the child is in puberty.

☑ Remember that cerebral injury, such as hypoxic-ischaemic encephalopathy during the neonatal period or hydrocephalus may cause PP later on or delayed puberty.

☑ PPP is either an isolated breast development (precocious thelarche) or sexual hair appearance (precocious adrenarche) without other signs of puberty occurring before the age of 8 years in girls and 9 years in boys. The condition is usually benign, non-progressive or very slowly progressive.

☑ In precocious thelarche (which usually occurs in toddlers), the nipple is characteristically pale, immature, thin and transparent. In contrast, the breasts of genuine PP are mature with prominent nipple and dark areola indicating high circulating oestrogen.

☑ The main differentiating feature between central (hypothalamic) and adrenal causes is that the PP is always isosexual in the former and testes remain small in the latter cause.

- Low-dose radiation of the brain has a high risk of inducing PP in girls, while high-dose may induce PP in both sexes.
- Hypothyroidism can cause PP; children are, however, short and the growth velocity is decreased.
- Growth acceleration and advanced bone age (wrist X-ray) favour true PP against PPP.
- A child with precocious thelarche or adrenarche needs careful evaluation, as these cannot often be easily and definitely differentiated from true PP.
- Full investigation, including imaging of the central nervous system and abdomen, should be carried out for all children with PP who have progressive signs of puberty, are younger than 6 years, with neurological signs or if the diagnosis is uncertain.

Red flags

- In any child with PP, careful search of the skin is essential: café-au-lait maculae with smooth border suggest NF-1; while larger café-au-lait patches with irregular outline is consistent with McCune–Albright syndrome (polyostotic fibrous dysplasia of bone, and ovarian cysts).
- Beware that in many normal girls thelarche is asymmetric and the breast nodule may be tender and sensitive to friction.
- Beware that children with hypothalamic lesion may present with diabetes insipidus (polydipsia, polyuria), hyperthermia, obesity or loss of weight, or inappropriate crying or laughter.
- Beware that PP may put girls at high risk of sexual abuse and psychological trauma from teasing and bullying.
- In a child with central PP, hypothalamic hamartoma (ectopically neural tissue secreting pulse GnRH) is probably the most common identifiable lesion causing PP. In addition to an urgent request for brain MRI, careful examination of visual acuity, visual fields, extraocular movements and eye fundi is essential.

NOTES:

Hair and nails

Alopecia (hair loss)

Excessive body hair

Itchy scalp

Abnormal nails

ALOPECIA (HAIR LOSS)

The clinician overview

Hair, derived from the epidermis, develops around the third to fourth month of the fetal life. At birth, the number of hair follicles on the scalp (about a million) and on other parts of the body (about 4 million) stabilises, and no more follicles are developed. The hair cycle consists of a growing phase of hair (anagen), which lasts about 3 months and constitutes about 90% of the total hair, and a resting phase (telogen), which also lasts about 3 months. Alopecia is not very common in children but is usually traumatic for the child and their parents. Common age is 5–12 years. It may occur in patches (areata), on the entire scalp (totalis) or over the entire body (universalis). Alopecia may also be scarring or non-scarring. Alopecia areata is the most common type of alopecia, affecting 1%–2% of the world's population. In children the prognosis is good; some 80%–90% will experience regrowth of their hair within a year. Hypotrichosis indicates deficient hair growth.

Possible diagnoses

INFANTS
Common

- ☑ Normal (after lanugo hair shedding)
- ☑ Pressure alopecia
- ☑ Seborrhoeic dermatitis
- ☑ Hidrotic ectodermal dysplasia
- ☑ Congenital alopecia (autosomal recessive)

Rare

- ☑ Syndrome (e.g. Menkes' kinky hair)
- ☑ Telogen effluvium
- ☑ Child abuse
- ☑ Endocrine (e.g. hypothyroidism, hypopituitarism)
- ☑ Toxic alopecia
- ☑ Genetic alopecia (autosomal dominant)
- ☑ Syndrome (e.g. Hallermann–Streiff)
- ☑ Metabolic (e.g. homocystinuria, aciduria)

CHILDREN

- ☑ Alopecia areata (also totalis, universalis)
- ☑ Tinea capitis
- ☑ Nutritional (e.g. marasmus, zinc deficiency)
- ☑ Drugs (e.g. cytotoxic, anticoagulants)
- ☑ Trauma (traction alopecia, compulsive pulling)

- ☑ Child abuse
- ☑ Cicatrical alopecia (e.g. systemic lupus erythematosus, lichen planus)
- ☑ Infection (e.g. typhoid fever, syphilis)

Differential diagnosis at a glance

	Alopecia areata	Tinea capitis	Nutritional	Drugs	Trauma
Patchy	Yes	Yes	Possible	Possible	Yes
Scalp otherwise normal	Yes	No	Possible	Yes	Yes
Pruritus	No	Yes	No	No	No
Diagnosis by Wood's light	No	Yes	No	No	No
Infancy	No	Possible	Possible	Possible	No

Recommended investigations

***   Wood's light confirms tinea infection. Microscopic examination of scrapings with potassium hydroxide is also diagnostic of the infection.

***   TFTs, FSH, LH, prolactin to screen for endocrine diseases.

***   Levels of zinc, iron, total protein and fractions for nutritional causes.

**   Autoimmune screen (e.g. ANA) for cases of alopecia areata.

***   Investigations to exclude possible metabolic causes (e.g. homocystinuria) if clinically indicated.

TOP TIPS

- Patchy alopecia on the occipital or temporal area in a baby is very common and is usually due to pressure from sleeping most of the time on that area. Sweating (e.g. due to warm clothes) causes rubbing and worsens the condition.
- When examining a child with alopecia, find out whether it is diffuse or patchy, inflammatory or non-inflammatory, scarring or non-scarring. This will help with the differential diagnosis.
- Diagnostic sign for alopecia areata is 'exclamation mark' hairs, which are 1–2 mm in length, tapered at the attached end and seen at the periphery of new bald patches.
- Nutritional causes of alopecia in developing countries are common, e.g. marasmus (protein-calorie deficiency) seen often during the first year of life, and kwashiorkor (protein deficiency).
- We should differentiate among anagen effluvium (toxic alopecia resulting from, for example, radiation, chemotherapy, thallium), traction alopecia (trauma to hair follicles resulting from traction by tight headbands, ponytails, rollers, curlers) and trichotillomania (which may be a benign habit or as part of obsessive–compulsive disorder (OCD)).
- Telogen effluvium (diffuse form of hair loss) may occur following stress or medications (e.g. childbirth, febrile illness, surgery, severe weight loss, discontinuation of high dose of steroids), or may occur in infancy as an incomplete alopecia. Parents can be reassured that hair will regrow in about 6 months' time.

- In any case of alopecia, tinea capitis has to be excluded. Wood's light is diagnostic.
- If the onset of alopecia areata occurs in early childhood and the alopecia is extensive, with loss of eyebrows and lashes, the prognosis is bad. In the absence of these risk factors parents and children can be reassured but it may take 1 year for the hair to regrow.
- Any child with alopecia areata should be examined and investigated for other autoimmune disorders such as vitiligo, coeliac disease, diabetes, Addison's disease. Good history is essential.
- Trauma caused by traction of hair follicles (from tight braids or ponytails) is common in girls of school age. They should be encouraged to avoid devices that cause trauma to hair.
- In trichotillomania (compulsive pulling of hair), children cannot resist the impulse of pulling at their hair. Although it can sometimes be a benign habit disorder, many children suffer from emotional stress and OCD, and the need to refer them for psychiatric consultation is indicated.

- Beware alopecia caused by child abuse. The hairs are typically broken at various lengths. Examine the skin carefully for other signs of abuse such as bruises.

NOTES:

EXCESSIVE BODY HAIR

The clinician overview

Vellus hair is fine, soft and non-pigmented, and covers most of the body before puberty. Terminal hair, in contrast, is coarse, curly and pigmented. Pubertal androgens promote the conversion from vellus to terminal hair. Hair growth in excess of what is expected for age, sex and ethnicity is termed hirsuitism or hypertrichosis. The condition is not common in children. It may be localised or generalised, transient or permanent. While hypertrichosis indicates non-androgenic excessive vellus hair growth in areas not usually hairy, hirsuitism is an androgen-dependent male pattern of hair growth usually in women. The most common cause of hypertrichosis or hirsuitism is racial or familial, which is frequent in people from the Mediterranean area and Indian subcontinent. In this country, the most common cause of hirsuitism is polycystic ovary syndrome (POS). Among the most important endocrine causes are congenital adrenal hyperplasia (CAH) and Cushing's syndrome.

Possible diagnoses

INFANTS
Common
- Lanugo hair (racial)
- Drugs
- Endocrine (e.g. CAH)
- Congenital pigmented hairy nevus
- Congenital melanocytic nevus

Rare
- Congenital hypertrichosis
- Ambras syndrome
- Cornelia de Lange syndrome
- Fetal hydantoin syndrome
- Localised

CHILDREN

- Racial and familial hypertrichosis or hirsuitism
- Drugs (e.g. steroids, phenytoin, cyclosporine, minoxidil)
- Endocrine causes (e.g. Cushing's syndrome, CAH, adrenal tumour)
- PCOS
- Malnutrition, including anorexia nervosa

- Hyperprolactinaemia
- Pituitary adenoma
- Cornelia de Lange syndrome
- Porphyria cutanae tarda
- Sertoli-Leydig cell tumour
- Granulosa-theca cell tumour

- ☑ Congenital terminal hypertrichosis with gingival hyperplasia
- ☑ Idiopathic hirsuitism
- ☑ Paraneoplastic syndrome

Differential diagnosis at a glance

	Racial and familial	Drugs	Endocrine causes	PCOS	Malnutrition
The only sign	Yes	Possible	Possible	No	No
Signs of masculinisation	No	Possible	Possible	Yes	No
Likely non-White race	Yes	No	No	No	Possible
Underweight	No	No	Possible	No	Yes
Present at birth	Yes	No	Possible	No	No

Recommended investigations

***   Urine porphyrins: for porphyria; 24-hour collection for cortisol levels.

***   U&E: for salt-losing CAH.

***   Serum testosterone, DHEAS, LH, FSH: raised in PCOS and tumour.

***   Serum 17-hydroxyprogesterone, DHEAS will confirm CAH.

***   Serum prolactin to diagnose hyperprolactinaemia.

***   TFTs for thyroid diseases.

***   Ultrasound scan for PCOS and CAH; MRI is often required, particularly if hormonal studies have been inconclusive, and for pituitary adenoma, adrenal and ovarian cysts or tumours.

TOP TIPS

- ☑ Although the term hirsuitism is mostly used in women, remember that hirsuitism in pre-pubertal children occurs equally in both sexes, and is an important sign of precocious puberty.
- ☑ Excessive hair growth is mostly racial and familial, so investigation is often not required.
- ☑ The benign form of hirsuitism is characterised by its pubertal onset and slow progression over many years. PCOS is an example of this and affects 5%–10% of women of reproductive age.
- ☑ Children with PCOS usually present at the time of puberty with menstrual disturbances, hirsuitism and being overweight.

- Hirsuitism, congenital or acquired, is caused by excessive androgen. Patients often have deepening of the voice, acne, irregular menstruation and a masculine body.
- Ultrasonography has an important role to play in this condition, e.g. determining uterus and ovaries in masculine signs of CAH, identification of multicystic ovaries (pearl necklace) in PCOS and detecting ovarian and adrenal tumours.
- Although most causes of hypertrichosis are benign, the condition often causes disfigurement and psychological trauma; referral to a dermatologist is indicated to obtain the most adequate therapy.

Red flags

- Paraneoplastic syndrome is a rare disorder of a wide variety of clinical pictures (e.g. myasthenic syndrome with lung cancer) that occur at sites distant from the tumour.
- Any acute and/or severe hirsuitism requires investigation to exclude serious underlying causes such as tumour of the ovary or adrenal cortex.
- Beware that, while high levels of testosterone with normal DHEAS indicates that the ovaries are producing the androgens, high levels of testosterone with high DHEAS indicates that the adrenals are producing the androgen.
- Hypertrichosis must be distinguished from hirsuitism causing virilisation; the latter is associated with acne, increased muscle bulk, deepening of the voice and clitoromegaly.
- In CAH, steroidogenesis has taken place in utero, therefore signs of masculinisation (enlarged and fused clitoris, resembling a penis and labial fusion) are present at birth. A mistaken diagnosis of cryptorchidism and hypospadias is often made.

NOTES:

ITCHY SCALP

The clinician overview

Itchy scalp is common and caused by a variety of conditions including dry skin (xerosis), eczema, pediculosis, scabies, fungal and bacterial infections, psoriasis and lichen planus. Of the three types of lice, *Pediculus humanus capitis*, *corporis* and *pubis*, pediculosis capitis is the most common and important type. The diagnosis is easy in the vast majority of cases and should be made by thorough examination of the scalp before considering any treatment.

Possible diagnoses

INFANTS

Common
- Excessive wrapping, high ambient temperature
- Scabies
- Pediculosis capitis
- Cholestasis
- Atopic dermatitis

Rare
- Poor hygiene including neglect
- Impetigo
- HIV
- Drugs (e.g. iron, zinc)
- Acute viral infection (e.g. varicella)

CHILDREN

- Pediculosis capitis
- Scabies
- Atopic dermatitis
- Dry skin (xerosis)
- Tinea capitis

- Poor hygiene
- Contact dermatitis
- Acne vulgaris
- Psoriasis
- Folliculitis
- Impetigo
- Discoid lupus
- Lichen simplex (neurogenic excoriation)
- Acute viral infection such as varicella
- Papular urticaria
- Obstructive jaundice (liver disease)
- Drugs (e.g. iron and zinc preparations, opioids)
- Dermatitis herpetiformis

Differential diagnosis at a glance

	Pediculosis capitis	Scabies	Atopic dermatitis	Dry skin	Tinea capitis
Visible ova	Yes	No	No	No	No
Skin lesions elsewhere	No	Possible	Yes	Possible	No
Hair growth normal	Yes	Yes	Yes	Yes	No
Associated fever and lymphadenopathy	Possible	Possible	Possible	No	Possible
Pustules	Possible	Possible	Possible	No	Possible

Recommended investigations

** Wood's light and/or microscopy of the hair and scalp (with potassium hydrochloride preparation of scrapings) can confirm fungal infection.

** Microscopic identification of mites from their burrows in cases of scabies.

** Gram stain and culture from the follicular orifice to identify the bacteria in folliculitis.

TOP TIPS

☑ In infants, warm wrapping and warm ambient temperature are common causes of restlessness, sweating and pruritis.

☑ Remember that poor hygiene is often the underlying cause of many conditions with scalp itching, such as pediculosis. Examination of the child may confirm other areas of their body with poor hygiene.

☑ Note that, while bullae, pustules and superimposed dermatitis of the skin and scalp dominate the clinical picture in infants with scabies, in older children, small papules and vesicles localised in the interdigital space and wrist flexors are seen.

☑ Wood's light is a very useful tool to have: blue-green fluorescence is detectable in the hair shaft infected by fungal infection. Tinea versicolour have golden fluorescence. A dark room is needed.

☑ As lice and ova (nits) are often hard to see in fair hair, the best way to identify lice is to comb the hair properly with a louse comb, preferably from the hairs behind the ears and back of the neck.

☑ Common cause of scalp pruritis is contact dermatitis due to the use of soaps, shampoo and other hair products, particularly those that contain alcohol.

☑ Although pruritic patchy alopecia is often caused by alopecia areata or tinea capitis, discoid lupus erythematosus and secondary syphilis should be considered in the differential diagnosis.

☑ For intense itching, local treatment of the scalp is often insufficient; oral antihistamine is needed.

Red flags

- ☑ In children with impaired immunity (e.g. HIV) or receiving immunosuppressive drugs including steroids, widespread and highly contagious rash with thick scaling may occur (Norwegian scabies). The nails become thickened and dystrophic with subungual debris densely populated by mites.
- ☑ Fever, regional lymphadenopathy and widespread pustules causing bacterial infection often complicate pediculosis, tinea capitis and scalp dermatitis. It is essential to search for the cause of this inflammatory response.
- ☑ Remember that some drugs (e.g. iron, zinc, opioids) can directly cause itching; other drugs (e.g. chlorpromazine) may indirectly cause itching by causing obstructive jaundice.
- ☑ If the cause of scalp itching is not straightforward, depression and anxiety may be the cause.

NOTES:

ABNORMAL NAILS

The clinician overview

Abnormal nails may occur as a result of generalised skin disease, skin disease confined to the nails, systemic disease, drugs, fungal or bacterial infection or tumour. It is important to distinguish between congenital and acquired abnormalities. The appearance of the nails may suggest an underlying systemic disease. For example, absent nails (anonychia) or small nails may occur in epidermolysis bullosa, acrodermatitis enteropathica, incontinentia pigmenti or nail–patella syndrome. Other nail abnormalities associated with systemic diseases include clubbing, seen in patients with cyanotic congenital heart, pulmonary (e.g. cystic fibrosis) and inflammatory bowel diseases. Splinter haemorrhage is an important clue to subacute bacterial endocarditis.

Possible diagnoses

INFANTS
Common
- Koilonychia (nail flattening and concavity = spoon-shaped)
- Paronychial inflammation (bacterial or fungal infection)
- Small or absent nails
- Trauma
- Atopic dermatitis

Rare
- Effect of drugs
- Pachyonychia congenita
- Nail–patella syndrome

CHILDREN
- Clubbing
- Koilonychia
- Paronychial inflammation
- Onycholysis (separation of nail plate from the distal nail bed)
- Onychomycosis (fungal infection)

- Effect of drugs (e.g. chloroquine, bleomycin)
- Psoriatic nails
- Small or absent nails
- Leukonychia
- Norwegian scabies (*see* Itchy scalp section)
- Ingrown nails
- Tumour (e.g. periungual fibroma, subungual melanoma)
- Nail–patella syndrome
- Yellow nail syndrome

- ☑ Drugs (e.g. indomethacin, vincristine)
- ☑ Longitudinal or transverse ridges
- ☑ Beau's lines (caused by, e.g., arsenic poisoning)

Differential diagnosis at a glance

	Clubbing	Koilonychia	Paronychial inflammation	Onycholysis	Onychomycosis
May be normal	Yes	Yes	No	No	No
May be painful	No	No	Yes	Possible	Possible
Skin lesions elsewhere	No	No	Possible	Possible	No
Inherited	Possible	Possible	No	Possible	No
Acute history	No	No	Yes	Possible	Possible

Recommended investigations

*** FBC and serum ferritin in spoon-shaped nails to exclude anaemia.

** Throat swab for culture and ASO titre in cases of acute psoriasis (guttate form).

** Wood's light and microscopy of culture in fungal infection.

TOP TIPS

- ☑ Koilonychia (spoon-shaped nails) can be normal during the first 2 years of life or there is an underlying iron-deficiency anaemia (Plummer–Vinson syndrome). The normal koilonychia corrects itself later after the age of 2 years.
- ☑ Pachyonychia congenita is an autosomal dominant trait associated with hypertrophic nail dystrophy (pachyonychia); it often leads to paronychia, nail loss and keratoderma.
- ☑ Small or absent nails may occur in association with nail–patella syndrome, in which the nail size is reduced by 30%–50%. This is an autosomal dominant disease with small and unstable patella.
- ☑ Paronychial inflammation may occur after prolonged immersion in water, which may occur with prolonged thumb- or finger-sucking.
- ☑ Nail involvement is a valuable diagnostic sign in psoriasis: pitting of the nail plate, onycholysis and yellow-brown subungual discolouration of the nails.
- ☑ Remember that the nail plate is relatively pliable and thin during the first 1–2 years of life; thus, spoon-shaped nails (koilonychia) at this age can be normal. Don't mistake them as pathological.

- In paediatrics, nail clubbing is the most important of all nail abnormalities. It is often seen in children with cystic fibrosis, inflammatory bowel diseases, cyanotic congenital heart diseases, bronchiectasis, as well as in healthy people (idiopathic or inherited).
- Both flattening and concavity (koilonychia) and white opacity of the nails (leukonychia) may harbour an underlying disease such as anaemia.
- Onycholysis is often due to trauma or psoriasis; in their absence, hyperthyroidism should be considered in the differential diagnosis.
- Although subungual splinter haemorrhage (red-brown longitudinal lines resulting from capillary leakage) may occur as a result of trauma or psoriasis, they are a very important clue to subacute bacterial endocarditis. The presence of cardiac murmur and fever clinch the diagnosis.

NOTES:

Neck

Sore throat and mouth

Hoarseness and changes of voice

Stridor

Neck lumps

Stiff and wry neck

Swallowing difficulty (dysphagia)

SORE THROAT AND MOUTH

The clinician overview

Sore throat and mouth are usually due to inflammatory or infective causes. The most common cause in young children is by far a viral upper respiratory tract infection (URTI). An infection rate of 6–8 infections a year is very common. Higher incidence is found in infants and children who attend daycare and whose siblings attend daycare or school. Acute tonsillopharyngitis refers to the tonsilo-pharynx as the principal site of the inflammatory process. Viruses (e.g. adenoviruses, Epstein–Barr viruses (EBV)) and bacteria (e.g. group A β-haemolytic streptococci (GAHS)) have overlapping symptoms and signs, and clinically they are often indistinguishable from one another. Tonsillopharyngitis is uncommon in children younger than 1 year of age; it peaks at the age of 4–7 years and continues throughout later childhood. Examination of the mouth should include the gingiva, buccal mucosa, tongue, teeth, hard and soft palate and posterior pharyngeal wall.

Possible diagnoses

INFANTS
Common
- ☑ Viral URTI
- ☑ Herpetic gingivostomatitis
- ☑ Oropharyngeal thrush
- ☑ Herpangina
- ☑ Any mouth ulceration (*see* Oral chapter)

Rare
- ☑ Neutropenia causing mouth ulceration
- ☑ Trauma
- ☑ Diphtheria

CHILDREN
- ☑ Viral URTI (viral tonsillopharyngitis)
- ☑ Bacterial tonsillopharyngitis (e.g. GAHS)
- ☑ Glandular fever (GF)
- ☑ Herpetic gingivostomatitis (herpes virus)
- ☑ Herpangina (coxsakievirus)

- ☑ Peritonsillar abscess/retropharyngeal abscess
- ☑ Dental pain
- ☑ Kawasaki's disease
- ☑ Scarlet fever
- ☑ Immunodeficiency (e.g. HIV infection)
- ☑ Leukopenia/neutropenia
- ☑ Epiglottitis
- ☑ Gonococcal pharyngitis
- ☑ Psychogenic (globus hystericus)
- ☑ Diphtheria

☑ Drugs (e.g. marijuana)
☑ Oropharyngeal thrush
☑ Aphthous ulceration

Differential diagnosis at a glance

	Viral URTI	Bacterial tonsillopharyngitis	GF	Herpetic gingivostomatitis	Herpangina
Gingival lesions	No	No	No	Yes	No
Lymphadenopathy	Possible	Possible	Yes	Possible	No
Response to antibiotics	No	Yes	No	No	No
Vesicles and ulcers	No	No	No	Yes	Yes
Exudate on tonsils	Possible	Yes	Yes	No	Possible

Recommended investigations

** FBC may show leukocytosis in bacterial infection, lymphocytosis in GF.

** An ASO-titre with fourfold increase in 1–2 weeks is the only diagnostic test for streptococcal infection.

*** Monospot is useful to diagnose GF (sensitive in about 90%; specific in 95%). IgM for EBV is positive in almost 100%. PCR for detection of EBV is now in routine use to aid diagnosis.

** Throat swab to culture group A-streptococci may be useful.

TOP TIPS

☑ While young children should be examined sitting restrained in the parent's lap, most older children are cooperative in opening their mouth without the use of a tongue depressor.

☑ The majority of tonsillopharyngitis are caused by viral infections in association with an URTI; antibiotics, therefore, are not indicated in the majority of cases.

☑ The main indication in antibiotic therapy of bacterial pharyngitis is not only to treat the symptoms but also to prevent complications, e.g. peritonsillar abscess, rheumatic fever (RF) and glomerulonephritis (GN).

☑ Remember that colonisation with GAHS occurs in 10%–20% of normal school-age children. They are not at risk of developing RF or GN. Therefore, a throat swab in acute illness is of limited value.

☑ In contrast to herpetic stomatitis caused by herpes virus, which has lesions on the gingiva, in herpangina (caused by coxsackievirus), there are discrete punctuate vesicles, surrounded by erythematous rings on the soft palate, anterior pillars and uvula and tonsils.

- Dental diseases are often not considered in the physical examination of the mouth. Tapping on the tooth's surface may be painful due to an abscess that is the cause of the sore mouth.
- When there is a membrane exudate on the tonsils, mononucleosis is likely, and antibiotics should not be administered to prevent skin eruption. Diphtheria may cause similar membrane exudate but this infection is now exceedingly rare.

Red flags

- Indication for tonsillectomy because of their large size is obsolete, and a referral for that is inappropriate. It is normal for early school-age children to have large tonsils. The absolute indication for tonsillectomy is the removal of tumour or airway obstruction (causing sleep apnoea).
- Beware that agranulocytosis may present with a sore throat as the first sign of the disease.
- Beware rare but important infections of peritonsillar or retropharyngeal abscess. Following improved symptoms of the primary infection (tonsillitis), there is an abrupt onset of high fever, with severe sore throat and distress. An urgent consultation with an ENT specialist is essential.
- Many systemic diseases (e.g. Crohn's disease) manifest as ulcers in the oral cavity, which present subjectively as a sore throat. Look for an underlying disease for any unexplained mouth ulcers.
- Consider immunosuppression, e.g. HIV, in any child older than a neonate with candida infection.

NOTES:

HOARSENESS AND CHANGES OF VOICE

The clinician overview

Hoarseness and stridor occur subsequent to an acute upper airway obstruction, commonly in association with a viral URTI (particularly parainfluenza type B viruses) or without it (spasmodic croup). Symptoms at first are mild and transient and recovery within a few days is usually the rule. More severe degrees of obstruction produce rapidly progressive respiratory distress with worsening cough, irritability, restlessness, nasal flaring and subcostal and intercostal recession. Such an obstruction may be caused by an URTI (viral croup or laryngotracheobronchitis), corynebacterium diphtheria (causing diphtheritic croup), staphylococcal aureus (causing bacterial tracheitis) or H. influenzae type B (causing epiglottitis). The obstruction is more serious in infants and young children than in older children because of the smaller airway. Persistent hoarseness suggests cord paralysis or tumours.

Possible diagnoses

INFANTS
Common
- Trauma to vocal cords
- Excessive crying
- Prolonged ventilation (vocal nodule)
- Central nervous system (CNS) disease (Chiari's malformation)
- Viral laryngotracheobronchitis

Rare
- Benign tumour (haemangioma)
- Cri-du-chat syndrome (5p deletion)

CHILDREN
- Viral croup (laryngotracheobronchitis)
- Spasmodic croup
- Angioedema
- Overuse of the voice (e.g. at athletic events)
- Tumour (e.g. papilloma, haemangioma, nodule)

- Aspiration of foreign body
- Bacterial tracheitis (staphylococcal infection)
- Epiglottitis
- Infectious mononucleosis
- Hypothyroidism
- Recurrent laryngeal nerve palsy (postoperative)
- Diphtheritic croup

- Measles croup
- Heavy cigarette smoking
- Retropharyngeal or peritonsillar abscess
- Laryngeal abscess
- Hypocalcaemic tetany

Differential diagnosis at a glance

	Viral croup	Spasmodic croup	Angioedema	Overuse of the voice	Tumour
Fever	Possible	No	No	No	No
Proceeded by URTI	Yes	No	No	No	No
Onset at night	Yes	Yes	No	No	No
Ill-looking	Possible	No	Yes	No	Possible
Stridor	Yes	Yes	Possible	Possible	Possible

Recommended investigations

Most cases of acute hoarseness and stridor do not need any investigation.

***   TFT to exclude hypothyroidism.

***   Serum calcium to confirm hypocalcaemia.

***   BC is indicated in suspected cases of epiglottitis.

**   Chest X-ray may diagnose vascular ring or aspiration. Upper airway X-ray to evaluate possible retropharyngeal or peritonsillar abscess.

***   Direct laryngoscopy to diagnose laryngeal node (post-ventilation), haemangiomas and unilateral or bilateral paralysis of the vocal cord.

**   CT scan or MRI of the head to diagnose Chiari's malformation.

TOP TIPS

- Laryngeal injury may occur subsequent to birth trauma (e.g. forceps delivery) and results in unilateral vocal cord paralysis (usually left side) producing hoarseness with mild stridor. Bilateral paralysis of the vocal cord also causes dyspnoea.
- Some congenital CNS diseases, such as Chiari's malformation, can produce unilateral or bilateral laryngeal nerve paralysis. Hoarseness, stridor and dyspnoea are the usual symptoms.
- The prognosis of post-ventilation aphonia or hoarseness is good and recovery is expected.
- The prognosis of viral and spasmodic croup is excellent. Only about 1%–2% of children with viral croup have severe symptoms requiring intensive care and intubation.
- In epiglottitis the voice is actually not hoarse, but muffled, because vocal cords are not affected.

- Symptoms of laryngotracheobronchitis do not usually continue for more than a few days. Persistent hoarseness requires laryngoscopy to detect the cause.

Red flags

- A child with 'croup' who rapidly becomes unwell with high fever has developed extension of the infection into the respiratory tract, bacterial tracheitis as a complication of the viral croup or bacterial epiglottitis.
- Birth trauma can cause unilateral or bilateral vocal cord paralysis, which may lead to recurrent pneumonia caused by recurrent aspiration.
- In cases of viral croup or epiglottitis, throat inspection, including the use of a tongue depressor, may result in sudden cardiorespiratory arrest and therefore should be omitted.
- Children with suspected epiglottitis must be immediately admitted. Consultation with an ENT specialist and anaesthetist should urgently be sought.
- In contrast to lower respiratory tract obstruction, children with croup do not usually have hypoxia (normal oxygen saturation); if hypoxia is detected, the condition is likely to be severe.
- A young child (aged from 6 months to 2 years) with sudden choking, coughing with or without stridor or hoarseness should be suspected of having a foreign body.
- In a severe allergic reaction, sudden onset of angioedema of the subglottic areas may occur, causing sudden stridor and respiratory distress. Adrenaline injection is life-saving.
- Papilloma is the most common tumour of the larynx. Although usually benign and often regressing at the time of puberty, it can extend into the lower airways and lungs, causing a serious disease.

NOTES:

STRIDOR

The clinician overview

Stridor is a harsh inspiratory sound caused by extrathoracic airway obstruction. It is predominately inspiratory due to obstruction in the subglottic area or trachea down to the thoracic inlet. Stridor can occur in both phases of respiration when the obstruction is severe. Most cases of acute stridor are due to laryngotracheobronchitis (croup) mainly caused by parainfluenza viruses type B, respiratory syncytial virus (RSV), adenoviruses, influenza viruses A and B, measles virus and mycoplasma pneumoniae. The infection usually produces inflammation affecting the larynx, trachea, bronchi and, sometimes, pulmonary parenchyma. The onset is usually with an upper respiratory tract infection, followed by barking cough, hoarseness and varying degrees of respiratory distress. Persistent stridor commencing in the first few weeks of life is mostly caused by laryngomalacia as a result of collapse of the supraglottic structure during inspiration. A child with laryngomalacia has a normal cry (no hoarse voice) and no cough.

Possible diagnoses

INFANTS
Common
- Birth trauma
- Laryngomalacia
- Haemangioma
- Croup
- Post-ventilation nodule

Rare
- Vascular ring
- Bifid epiglottis
- Laryngeal web
- Diphtheritic croup
- Laryngo-tracheo-oesphageal cleft

CHILDREN

- Croup (laryngotracheobronchitis)
- Spasmodic croup
- Bacterial tracheitis
- Laryngomalacia
- Angioneurotic oedema

- Epiglottitis
- Foreign body
- Measles croup
- Hypocalcaemia (tetany with laryngospasm)

Differential diagnosis at a glance

	Croup	Spasmodic croup	Bacterial tracheitis	Laryngomalacia	Angioneurotic oedema
Short history	Yes	Yes	Yes	No	Yes
Fever	Possible	No	Yes	No	No
Preceding URTI	Yes	No	Possible	No	No
Onset at night	Yes	Yes	No	No	No
Hoarseness	Yes	Yes	No	No	Possible

Recommended investigations

Most acute cases of croup do not require any investigation.
*** Serum calcium for suspected hypocalcaemic tetany.
*** Laryngoscopy is indicated by atypical features, e.g. feeding problems or worsening stridor.

TOP TIPS

◪ Laryngeal injury may occur subsequent to birth trauma (e.g. forceps delivery) or some congenital central nervous system (CNS) diseases (e.g. Chiari's malformation). These cause unilateral or bilateral vocal cord paralysis producing stridor hoarseness and dyspnoea.

◪ Determine whether the stridor is acute or chronic to narrow the diagnostic possibilities.

◪ The most important aspect of acute stridor is to differentiate between a life-threatening illness such as epiglottitis or foreign body and a relatively harmless croup caused by a viral infection.

◪ Nocturnal onset of acute stridor with barking cough and hoarseness is almost certainly a viral croup or spasmodic cough. Despite the frightening symptoms, the outcome is very good.

◪ Laryngomalacia is the most common cause of persistent stridor in infancy. It is caused by a soft tissue laxity above the vocal cords that collapses during inspiration. Parents can be reassured that recovery is expected aged 12–18 months, often even earlier. Another cause is tumour.

◪ Once the diagnosis of laryngomalacia is made, direct examination of the larynx is not indicated unless there are atypical features such as associated feeding problems or worsening stridor.

- Birth trauma and some CNS malformation can cause unilateral or bilateral vocal cord paralysis, which may lead to recurrent pneumonia caused by recurrent aspiration.
- A neonate with respiratory distress and severe stridor could have laryngeal web occurring between the vocal cords. Immediate diagnosis by direct laryngoscopy is required to prevent asphyxia. Laser treatment is frequently successful.
- A toxic-looking child with high fever and swallowing difficulty is having epiglottitis. Admit to intensive care unit, and consult an ENT specialist and an anaesthetist. Do not examine the throat as this could cause laryngeal spasm and respiratory obstruction.
- Do not diagnose laryngomalacia if there are signs of respiratory distress, apnoea or cyanotic episodes or failure to thrive. Referral and arrangement for laryngoscopy are indicated.
- In the absence of a viral respiratory tract infection, an acute stridor in a toddler may suggest foreign body. This is more likely if the history suggests sudden choking and coughing.
- Some children with croup (1%–2%) may present with increasing respiratory distress and worsening tachycardia. They will need intensive care and intubation.
- It is unusual for the common croup to have hypoxia (pulse oximeter below 92%). If present this would be an ominous sign requiring close monitoring.

NOTES:

NECK LUMPS

The clinician overview

Lumps in the neck are common and are usually benign. Of the many lumps found in the neck, cervical lymphadenopathy is the most common physical finding. It usually results from viral infection leaving behind small (< 1 cm), non-tender mobile lymph nodes, which are considered normal in children. Lymph nodes are not considered enlarged until their diameter exceeds 1 cm for cervical and axillary lymph nodes and 1.5 cm for inguinal lymph nodes. About one-third of neonates have palpable lymph nodes, usually smaller than 1 cm in diameter. They are commonly present in the inguinal area (due to the prevalence of infection of the nappy area) but may also be noted in the cervical or axillary region. Generalised lymphadenopathy indicates involvement of enlarged lymph nodes in more than two node regions. Pathological lymphadenopathy is suggested by abnormally large lymph nodes, which are tender, hard, matted together or fixed to the skin or underlying structures, or localised in the supraclavicular area.

Possible diagnoses

INFANTS
Common
- Lymphadenopathy
- Goitre
- Sternomastoid tumour
- Dermoid cyst
- Thyroglossal cyst

Rare
- Cystic hygroma
- Branchial cyst

CHILDREN

- Reactive lymphadenitis (due to local infection)
- Systemic infection (e.g. Kawasaki's disease, mononucleosis)
- Goitre
- Malignancy (e.g. lymphoma)
- Thyroglossal cyst

- Cystic hygroma (lymphatic malformation)
- TB lymphadenitis
- Pharyngeal pouch
- Lymphadenopathy of juvenile rheumatoid arthritis

Differential diagnosis at a glance

	Reactive lymphadenitis	Systemic disease	Goitre	Lymphoma	Thyroglossal cyst
Tender	Possible	Possible	No	No	No
Generalised	No	Yes	No	Possible	Yes
Moves with swallowing	No	No	Yes	No	Yes
Midline	No	No	Yes	No	Yes
Fixed to skin	No	No	No	Yes	No

Recommended investigations

** FBC and differential: leukocytosis suggests infection; atypical lymphocytes for mononucleosis; leukopenia for systemic lupus erythematosus; anaemia chronic infection or lymphoma.

** LFTs: abnormal in Epstein–Barr virus (EBV), cytomegalovirus (CMV).

** Monospot test or IgG for EBV.

*** Chest X-ray is first-line investigation and helpful in case of TB or lymphoma.

*** Ultrasound and/or MRI of the neck is useful to differentiate neck tumours.

*** Tuberculin skin test for suspected TB adenitis.

* Throat culture may be positive in bacterial lymphadenitis.

** Serum antibody studies for EBV, CMV, HIV, Bartonella (cat-scratch fever).

*** Needle aspiration for Gram stain and culture in suspected malignancy; excisional biopsy for TB.

TOP TIPS

☑ Remember that in a normal neonate, the thyroid cannot be felt; if it can be felt it is most likely enlarged. A soft thyroid can normally be palpated in older children.

☑ In any case with neck lumps, the size of the lump needs to be documented to monitor progress.

☑ Reactive lymphadenopathy is the most common reason for lumps in the neck. Parents usually fear the possibility of cancer and need to be reassured. Reactive lymphadenopathy may last months or years and may enlarge in response to another viral infection.

☑ Thyroglossal cyst, which develops from a remnant thyroglossal duct, is painless but becomes enlarged and tender if infected. Pathognomonic sign is its vertical movement on swallowing and tongue protrusion.

☑ Branchial cyst appears like an insignificant-looking papule on the side of the neck, off-centre (in contrast to thyroglossal cyst). Its surgical removal may be quite difficult to trace out its tract.

☑ The most common acquired goitre in children is Hashimoto's thyroiditis, which is associated with normal thyroid function or sometimes hypothyroidism.

◪ Generalised lymphadenopathy suggests systemic infection (e.g. AIDS, mononucleosis, toxoplasmosis), autoimmune disease (e.g. rheumatoid arthritis) or malignancy (e.g. leukaemia).

◪ Remember that lymphoma is often associated with B-symptoms: fever, weight loss, splenomegaly.

◪ Juvenile rheumatoid arthritis often presents with lymphadenopathy generalised, seen in systemic form (Still's disease) in association with fever, rash and hepatosplenomegaly.

◪ Midline neck masses are usually either thyroid or thyroglossal duct cyst (TDC). They can clinically be easily differentiated: while thyroid moves with swallowing, TDC moves upward when the tongue sticks out.

◪ Reactive lymphadenopathy should be differentiated from TB lymphadenitis. The latter appears as gradually enlarged nodes, firm but not hard, discrete and non-tender and usually unilateral.

Red flags

◪ Some lymph nodes are present in virtually any child; total absence of palpable lymph nodes suggests the possibility of immune deficiency such as agammaglobulinaemia.

◪ A 'thyroglossal cyst' should never be excised unless thyroid tissue is excluded. Such ectopic thyroid tissue is usually all the thyroid the child has.

◪ Beware that TB lymphadenitis is best diagnosed by excisional biopsy for histological and bacteriological confirmation and to exclude infection with non-tuberculous mycobacteria or cat-scratch fever. The biopsy, however, carries the risk of developing a fistula.

◪ Biopsy is indicated and urgent if the neck mass is associated with persistent or unexplained fever, night sweats, anorexia, weight loss or if the mass has progressively enlarged.

◪ A neck mass, matted or fixed to the underlying structures, should urgently be referred to the oncology specialist for suspected malignancy.

NOTES:

STIFF AND WRY NECK

The clinician overview

This symptom is extremely important because of the possibility of meningitis, and other serious bacterial infections such as pneumonia. It is a common complaint to both emergency and primary care clinicians. The term refers to abnormal position of the neck or restricted range of movement, usually associated with pain during passive and active neck movement. In infants, it is usually caused by shortening sternomastoid muscle following swelling formation (called sternomastoid tumour). In older children, an important cause is torticollis (wry neck), which is characterised by holding the neck tilted to one side with the chin rotated in the opposite direction, and meningism. Meningism is another important cause that always requires emergency evaluation. It is characterised by the presence of signs of neck stiffness in flexion position. The most common cause of meningism is meningeal irritation (meningitis, cerebral haemorrhage) but some cases may not have demonstrable meningeal infection. In contrast to torticollis, a child with meningism is usually ill-looking with fever. Cerebrospinal fluid examination is usually required to exclude meningitis.

Possible diagnoses

INFANTS
Common
- Muscular torticollis (sternomastoid tumour, CP)
- Sandifer's syndrome (GO reflux)
- Congenital abnormalities of cervical spine
- Klippel–Feil syndrome
- Meningitis

Rare
- Muscular cervical injury
- Pterygium colli

CHILDREN

- Meningitis
- Pneumonia (upper lobe pneumonia)
- Viral upper respiratory tract infection (URTI) with cervical lymphadenitis
- Acute torticollis (cervical muscle trauma)
- Neck injury (whiplash injury)

- Visual defects (nystagmus, superior oblique paresis)
- Dystonic drug reaction
- Hysteria
- Cervical spine infection
- Rheumatoid arthritis
- Polymyalgia rheumatica

- ☑ Tetanus
- ☑ Posterior fossa brain tumour
- ☑ Intracranial haemorrhage
- ☑ Retropharyngeal abscess
- ☑ Spasmus nutans

Differential diagnosis at a glance

	Meningitis	Pneumonia	Viral URTI with cervical lymphadenitis	Acute torticollis	Neck injury
Ill appearance	Yes	Yes	No	Possible	Yes
High fever	Yes	Yes	Possible	No	No
+ meningeal signs	Yes	No	No	No	No
Vomiting/headaches	Yes	Possible	No	Possible	No
History of trauma	No	No	No	Possible	Yes

Recommended investigations

***   FBC: leukocytosis suggest bacterial infection in meningitis and pneumonia.

***   Lumbar puncture (LP) is the most important test to exclude meningitis even in the presence of extra-neural infection.

***   In the presence of pulmonary symptoms, a chest X-ray is required to diagnose pneumonia.

***   Cervical X-ray to diagnose spinal abnormalities such as fusion of the vertebrae or injury.

**   Renal ultrasound scan to diagnose renal malformation (e.g. Klippel–Feil syndrome).

TOP TIPS

- ☑ Torticollis resulting from sternomastoid tumour is asymptomatic in the first few days of life. At 10–20 days, a mass is frequently felt in the muscle. The mass gradually disappears and the fibrous tissue contracts causing limited head motion and torticollis.
- ☑ Most cases of congenital torticollis are due to sternomastoid tumour, which is usually palpable on sternomastoid muscle. The torticollis responds to physiotherapy. Those infants with no history of birth trauma and no palpable mass should have anterio-posterior and lateral spine X-rays to exclude structural abnormalities before starting physiotherapy.
- ☑ Lymph nodes that enlarge with inflammation may never return to normal size; they remain as harmless palpable lumps for months and years.
- ☑ Although neck stiffness (nuchal rigidity) is a cardinal sign of meningeal irritation, including meningitis and haemorrhage, this sign is mainly beyond infancy.

- A child presenting with pain in the neck and mild neck stiffness following sleep may result from sleeping in an awkward position. Gentle active rotation and flexion is usually achievable.
- Children with torticollis and dystonic drug reaction look remarkably well despite the stiff neck, in contrast to those with meningitis or pneumonia.
- Not all pain on neck flexion means meningeal irritation; lymphadenitis and acute pharyngitis are more common causes.
- Drug history is of paramount importance to confirm a rare case of dystonic drug reaction (oculogyric crisis).

Red flags

- A child with Klippel–Feil malformation (short neck, fusion of the cervical vertebrae) has a high rate of renal malformations (40%).
- Any child with meningism should be considered as a case of meningitis until proved otherwise. Even if pneumonia is diagnosed, the case requires LP to confirm or exclude meningitis.
- The skin of a child with meningism should be carefully searched for any rash or petechiae in case of meningococcal disease.
- Meningitis, particularly meningococcal disease, may initially mimic virus-like illness. Within a few hours the disease can rapidly progress to septic shock, hypotension, disseminated intravascular coagulation and death.
- Although acquired torticollis is mostly due to minor cervical muscle trauma or an URTI, careful evaluation is essential to exclude serious conditions such as brain tumour or vertebral infection.

NOTES:

SWALLOWING DIFFICULTY (DYSPHAGIA)

The clinician overview

Swallowing is a complex mechanism involving some 50 muscle pairs (agonists and antagonists) to bring swallowed material to the stomach. Swallowing is developed in gestation as early as 20 weeks and is established at 33–34 weeks gestation. Dysphagia is defined as a difficulty in swallowing due to impaired transfer of fluids or food from the oral cavity to oesophagus (pre-oesophageal) and from oesophagus to stomach (oesophageal dysphagia). Causes of pre-oesophageal dysphagia include myasthenia gravis and pseudo-bulbar palsy. Causes of oesophageal dysphagia include stricture and oesophagitis. Dysphagia may include pain during swallowing (odynophagia), food sticking in the throat, the feeling of having a lump in the throat, and chest pain or discomfort during swallowing or regurgitation through the mouth or nose. In infants dysphagia may manifest as low interest in food, body stiffness or vomiting during feeding, unusually lengthy feeding, coughing or gagging during feeding.

Possible diagnoses

INFANTS
Common
- Extreme prematurity
- Oesophageal stenosis/atresia
- Any neonatal illness, e.g. RDS
- Cleft lip and palate
- Choanal stenosis/atresia

Rare
- Spasticity or muscular weakness (CP)
- Oesophagitis (GO reflux)
- Neuro-muscular (e.g. congenital myasthenia gravis (MG))
- Nasal obstruction (choanal stenosis/atresia)
- Prader–Willi syndrome

CHILDREN

- Oropharyngeal (e.g. tonsillitis, tonsillar abscess, epiglottitis)
- Spasticity (bulbar palsy)
- Globus hystericus
- Oesophagitis
- Collagen disease (e.g. dermatomyositis, scleroderma)

- Neuro-muscular (e.g. MG)
- Oesophageal stricture
- Oesophageal foreign body (FB)
- Oesophagitis (GO reflux, corrosive accidental ingestion)
- Scleroderma

☑ Vascular ring

☑ Spinal muscular atrophy or injury
☑ Eosinophilic oesophagitis
☑ Achalasia
☑ Vascular ring
☑ Lower oesophageal ring (Schatzki's ring)
☑ Plummer–Vinson syndrome (sideropenic dysphagia)
☑ Oesophageal diverticulum (pharyngeal or oesophageal)
☑ Drugs (potassium chloride, quinidine)

Differential diagnosis at a glance

	Oropharyngeal	Spasticity	Globus hystericus	Oesophagitis	Collagen vascular disease
Acute onset	Yes	No	Possible	Possible	No
Fever	No	No	No	No	Possible
Prior vomiting	Possible	Possible	No	Yes	Possible
Neuro signs	No	Yes	No	No	Possible
Symptom mild	Yes	No	Yes	Possible	Possible

Recommended investigations

**   Serum muscle enzymes elevated in dermatomyositis.
***   Chest X-ray, ultrasound scan for possible vascular ring.
***   Barium meal for any oesophageal cause of dysphagia, including external compression.
***   Oesophagoscopy to identify structural abnormalities or to obtain biopsy.
***   pH study to detect GO reflux.
***   Cine-fluoroscopy may detect oesophageal web and motor disorders such as achalasia.

TOP TIPS

☑ By term, the fetus is normally swallowing up to 500 mL of amniotic fluid each day. Inability to swallow fluid causes polyhydramnios (> 2000 mL in the third trimester).
☑ Note that intermittent dysphagia for both liquids and solids suggests a primary oesophageal motor disorder, whereas clearing an impacted bolus by vomiting suggests obstruction.
☑ A young patient who complains of having a lump in the throat or neck that is unrelated to swallowing is almost certainly having globus hystericus. This usually occurs in association with anxiety, stress or grief.

- Achalasia is a neurogenic oesophageal disorder of unknown aetiology that is characterised by absence of peristalsis during swallowing. The oesophagus empties poorly and food accumulates in the dilated atonic distal oesophagus. This can be demonstrated by barium meal.
- Unless the cause of the swallowing difficulty is easily established and acute, the management is the responsibility of an expert team including a speech-language therapist.
- Children with cerebral palsy who are at risk of aspiration and/or have naso-gastric tube feeding may be referred to a paediatric neurologist and surgeon for consideration of a gastrostomy.
- Although cleaning solutions accidentally ingested are the most common agents causing oesophageal stricture, certain drugs such as potassium chloride, tetracycline and quinidine can cause stricture if temporarily lodged in the oesophagus by motility disorder.

Red flags

- Untreated severe iron-deficiency anaemia can cause a thin mucosal membrane that grows across the lumen of the oesophagus.
- A neonate with excess secretions in the mouth, feeding difficulties and respiratory distress has oesophageal atresia until proven otherwise. Don't feed the baby until this diagnosis is excluded.
- Acute onset of dysphagia for both liquids and solids should always suggest the possibility of a FB obstructing the oesophagus.
- It is important to treat GO reflux before oesophagitis and stricture develop.
- Infants with swallowing difficulty who are fed by mouth are at high risk of aspiration, which leads to recurrent aspiration pneumonia.

NOTES:

Nose

Nasal discharge/blocked nose

Nosebleed (epistaxis)

NASAL DISCHARGE/ BLOCKED NOSE

The clinician overview

Nasal discharge and blockage are extremely common in children; causes and management should be familiar to all clinicians. By far the most common causes in practice are viral infectious rhinitis (more common in early years of childhood, when allergic rhinitis is uncommon), allergic rhinitis (more common in older children and adults) and adenoid hypertrophy. In neonates and young infants, nasal malformations such as congenital narrowing of the nasal passage, choanal atresia (incidence is one in 7000 live births) and stenosis have to be considered in the differential diagnosis, particularly if the symptoms are persistent. Although the vast majority of causes are benign and self-limiting, serious conditions include nasopharyngeal tumours, encephalocele and foreign body. In these conditions, discharge is usually purulent and foul smelling, with or without blood.

Possible diagnoses

INFANTS
Common
- Baby snuffles
- Viral infectious rhinitis
- Adenoid hypertrophy
- Congenital narrowing of nasal passages (excluding choanal atresia/stenosis)
- Choanal atresia/stenosis

Rare
- Allergic rhinitis
- Nasal septum deviation (birth trauma)
- Congenital syphilis
- Hypothyroidism
- Encephalocele
- Immotile ciliary syndrome
- Tumour
- CHARGE syndrome

CHILDREN
- Viral URTI
- Allergic rhinitis (AR)
- Adenoid hypertrophy
- Vasomotor rhinitis (VR)
- Nasal polyposis (cystic fibrosis (CF), allergy)

- Foreign body (occurring commonly in toddlers)
- Nasopharyngeal fibroma
- Deviated nasal septum
- Unilateral choanal atresia or stenosis
- Hypothyroidism
- Cocaine abuse
- Immotile ciliary syndrome
- Immunodeficiency
- Choanal stenosis

- ◪ Tumour
- ◪ Cerebrospinal fluid rhinorrhoea
- ◪ Rhinitis medicamentosa
- ◪ Encephalocele

Differential diagnosis at a glance

	Viral URTI	AR	Adenoid hypertrophy	VR	Nasal polyposis
Itching/sneezing	Possible	Yes	No	Possible	No
+ allergy tests	No	Yes	No	No	Possible
Infants affected	Yes	Possible	Yes	No	No
Other allergy symptoms	No	Possible	No	No	Possible
Prolonged symptoms	No	Yes	Yes	No	Yes

Recommended investigations

*   FBC: the presence of eosinophilia may suggest allergic rhinitis.

**   Allergy testing such as total IgE, skin prick testing and RASTs to identify possible allergens.

*   Sinus X-ray may identify sinus opacity suggestive of sinusitis or a mass.

*   Plain X-ray to identify adenoid hypertrophy.

***   CT scan is a better device than X-ray to diagnose sinusitis or the extent of tumour.

TOP TIPS

- ◪ Blocked nose in babies ('snuffles') is common due to the presence of mucous in a narrowed nasal passage. It is loud during feeding and sleep and disappears when the baby reaches 4–5 months; reassurance is the best medicine.
- ◪ Neonates are obligatory nasal breathers; therefore, those with bilateral choanal atresia present with severe respiratory distress and cyanosis that improves when the child cries.
- ◪ Unilateral choanal atresia or stenosis may be asymptomatic for many months and presents later as persistent unilateral nasal discharge or unilateral severe nasal obstruction.
- ◪ Diagnosis of atresia or stenosis is established by inability to pass a catheter through nostrils 3–4 cm into the nasopharynx.
- ◪ Remember that chronic nasal obstruction can be the cause rather than the result of sinusitis.
- ◪ Acute nasal obstruction with profuse watery discharge is suggestive of VR.

- Symptoms of VR resemble those of AR but with an allergic cause and eosinophils in the nasal secretion are absent, with nasal obstruction as the main symptom; itching and sneezing are minimal.
- It is easy for the clinician to diagnose polyps clinically. In contrast to the highly vascularised pink turbinate tissue, polyps are a grey, shiny, grape-looking mass present between the nasal turbinates and the septum.
- When adenoid hypertrophy is causing symptoms such as hearing impairment, restlessness at night or sleep apnoea, referral to an ENT specialist with consideration for adenoectomy is indicated.
- The presence of nasal polyps should lead clinicians to exclude CF, even in the absence of pulmonary or intestinal symptoms. Some 20%–25% of patients with CF have polyps.
- Overuse of over-the-counter medications (e.g. nasal spray or decongestants) may lead to rhinitis medicamentosa. Taking history should include what nasal medications have been used.

Red flags

- When choanal atresia is diagnosed, beware that 50% of those affected have other congenital anomalies (e.g. CHARGE syndrome).
- While a foul-smelling or blood-tinged unilateral discharge in a toddler suggests foreign body, a persistent bloody discharge always suggests tumour, including malignancy.
- Beware 'obstructive sleep apnoea' with chronic airway obstruction, including nasal obstruction, which can lead to chronic hypoxia, growth failure, pulmonary hypertension, right-sided heart failure and even death. Predisposing factors include adenotonsillar hypertrophy and trisomy-21.
- Beware of 'baby snuffles' due to the rare but important cause of congenital syphilis. Anaemia and splenomegaly are other findings.
- Some asthmatic children react with severe dyspnoea and nasal symptoms within 2 hours of aspirin ingestion. Look for evidence of nasal polyps and sinusitis to complete the 'aspirin triad', which consists of asthma, polyps and aspirin sensitivity.

NOTES:

NOSEBLEED (EPISTAXIS)

The clinician overview

Epistaxis is usually benign and self-limiting but often causes significant parental anxiety. It is a very common condition in paediatrics. About 30% of children aged under 5 years and over 50% aged 6–10 years experience at least one episode of epistaxis. Incidence is rare before 2 years of age and uncommon after puberty. The nasal mucosa of the nasal septum has a rich vascular supply arising from convergence of both internal and external carotid arteries (Kiesselbach's plexus). Epistaxis is classified, on the basis of bleeding site, into anterior and posterior. The majority of bleeds (about 90%) originate from the anterior caudal septum. This location, with its thin mucosa, is predisposed to trauma such as local irritation. Epistaxis may, however, be a sign of serious systemic disease such as coagulopathy or vascular disorder such as hereditary haemorrhagic telangiectasia (HHT). When dealing with severe epistaxis, assessment of the vital signs, airway and circulation stability are more important than the assessment of the bleeding itself.

Possible diagnoses

INFANTS
Common
- Coagulopathy (e.g. vitamin K deficiency)

Rare
- HIV
- Congenital vascular abnormalities (e.g. HHT)
- Choanal stenosis
- Idiopathic pulmonary haemosiderosis (haemoptysis presents as epistaxis)

CHILDREN
- Digital trauma (e.g. nose picking)
- Inflammation (hay fever, infectious rhinitis)
- Coagulopathy
- Foreign body
- Drugs (local decongestant, inhalants, cocaine, anticoagulant)

- Nasal polyps (e.g. cystic fibrosis, allergy)
- Chronic cocaine abuse
- Hypertension (very rare in children)
- Child abuse (physical abuse)
- Tumour (benign, such as haemangioma, or malignant)
- Juvenile nasal angiofibromatosis
- Ehlers–Danlos syndrome

◪ HHT (Osler–Weber–Rendu disease)
◪ Ataxia-telangiectasia

Differential diagnosis at a glance

	Digital trauma	Inflammation	Coagulopathy	Foreign body	Drugs
Severe epistaxis	Possible	No	Yes	No	No
Prior nasal obstruction	No	Yes	No	Yes	No
History suggests the diagnosis	Possible	Yes	Possible	No	Yes
Known recurrence	Possible	Possible	Possible	No	Possible
The only symptom	Possible	Possible	No	Yes	Possible

Recommended investigations

*** FBC: to check for Hb in case of massive bleeding; platelet count in case of thrombocytopenia.

*** Coagulation screens with PT (for vitamin K deficiency), PTT (to screen for haemophilia) and bleeding time for suspected von Willebrand's disease.

*** Further clotting studies if coagulation screens are abnormal.

*** Imaging with CT scan/MRI for severe and frequent epistaxis to exclude nasopharyngeal mass or pulmonary arteriovenous malformations in suspected case of HHT.

TOP TIPS

◪ Distinguishing between local and systemic causes of epistaxis is essential for the institution of appropriate therapy.

◪ A child with epistaxis should undergo thorough physical examination to exclude systemic disease such as coagulopathy, leukaemia or von Willebrand's disease. The parents will appreciate checking of the blood pressure as they may consider hypertension to be the cause.

◪ Ehlers–Danlos syndrome consists of a group of hereditary collagen disorders that share common features including joint hypermobility, skin hyperelasticity and fragility of the skin and blood vessels.

◪ In managing epistaxis, the nares should be compressed and the child kept as quiet as possible in an upright position with the head tilted forward to avoid blood trickling posteriorly in the pharynx.

◪ In adolescents with recurrent epistaxis and nasal ulcers, consider the possibility of cocaine use.

◪ Although lay people often associate epistaxis with hypertension, this is very rarely the case. Beware, however, that anxiety from having epistaxis may cause mild hypertension.

- Beware that epistaxis at night may cause swallowing of blood, causing haematemesis and/or melaena occurring next morning.
- At the initial evaluation, focus upon respiratory and haemodynamic stability of the patient rather than the bleeding.

Red flags

- Epistaxis is usually self-limiting and requires no investigation. Frequent and severe epistaxis should be investigated for an underlying disorder such as coagulopathy or tumour.
- Any epistaxis that occurs under the age of 2 years, particularly if severe, requires investigations to exclude systemic diseases such as blood dyscrasias or local tumour. Urgent referral to an ENT specialist is indicated.
- Epistaxis originating from the posterior bleeding site is uncommon in children and is usually profuse; inflammation or neoplasm should be excluded.
- Beware that massive epistaxis is often the first and only complaint of HHT before the appearance of the characteristic skin and mucosal membrane lesions, occurring in 80% of cases. Around 20% of patients have pulmonary arteriovenous malformations that may present as stroke due to embolic abscess.
- Juvenile nasal angiofibroma is a benign tumour of the nasopharynx that usually presents with nasal obstruction and epistaxis. The tumour may be mistaken as a nasal polyp.
- While a foul-smelling or blood-tinged unilateral discharge suggests foreign body, particularly in toddlers, a persistent bloody discharge always suggests tumour, including malignancy.

NOTES:

Oral

Mouth ulcers

Mouth bleeding

Bad breath (halitosis)

MOUTH ULCERS

The clinician overview

Mouth ulceration is common in children. It may be caused by trauma (physical or chemical), viral infections, aphthous ulcers, dermatological or haematopoietic disorders, gastrointestinal disease, nutritional deficiency, a side effect of drugs or periodic fever syndrome (such as periodic fever, aphthous stomatitis, pharyngitis and adenopathy = PFAPA). Most mouth ulcers in young children are caused by viral infection, such as acute herpetic gingivostomatitis (AHG), while aphthous ulcers are more common in older children and adults (affecting about 20% of the population), with a tendency to recur in contrast to AHG. Mouth ulcers are distressing and feeding is usually problematic.

Possible diagnoses

INFANTS
Common
- AHG
- Medications (e.g. chemotherapy, non-steroidal anti-inflammatory drugs)
- Trauma (including child abuse)
- Exanthem (e.g. varicella, measles)
- Neutropenia

Rare
- Periodic fever syndrome (e.g. PFAPA)
- Hand-foot-mouth disease

CHILDREN
- AHG
- Hand-foot-mouth disease
- Herpangina
- Trauma (including child abuse, chemical burns)
- Aphthous ulcers

- Other viral infections, e.g. varicella, cytomegalovirus
- Inflammatory bowel disease (Crohn's disease)
- Neutropenia (cyclic), aplastic anaemia
- Lichen planus
- Fungal infection
- Medications (e.g. chemotherapy)
- Histoplasmosis
- HIV infection
- Necrotising ulcerative gingivostomatitis (NUG)

- Periodic fever syndrome (e.g. PFAPA)
- Behçet's disease
- Systemic lupus erythematosus (SLE)
- Stevens–Johnson syndrome
- Vitamin deficiency (B_{12})
- Mouth cancer
- Reiter's syndrome (+ uveitis, conjunctivitis, arthritis)

Differential diagnosis at a glance

	AHG	Hand-foot-mouth disease	Herpangina	Trauma	Aphthous ulcers
Fever	Yes	Possible	Yes	No	No
Affects the gingiva	Yes	Possible	No	Possible	Possible
Size usually < 10 mm	Yes	Yes	Yes	Possible	Possible
Likely history of recurrence	No	No	No	Possible	Yes
Extra-oral sites	No	Yes	No	Possible	No

Recommended investigations

*** FBC: neutropenia in cyclic neutropenia, anaemia likely in Crohn's disease, leukopenia, anaemia and thrombocytopenia in SLE.

** CRP: elevated in bacterial infectious disease.

*** Serological tests for HIV infection.

*** Dark field microscopy from debris obtained from NUG lesions will demonstrate spirochetes.

** Scraping for culture in suspected fungal infection; if positive, tests for immunity are required.

TOP TIPS

- Benign aphthae tend to be small in size (< 1 cm) and self-limiting in duration (about 90% of cases), while large aphthae are often associated with more serious disorders such as HIV infection.
- Differentiating herpangina from AHG is usually easy: herpangina has more posterior lesions (tonsils, tonsillar pillars, uvula, pharyngeal wall and soft palate) while in AHG the lesions affect the cheeks, gingiva and tongue.

- Acute necrotising ulcerative gingivitis is rare in healthy children but may occur in association with malnutrition. It may mimic AHG, but dark field microscopy will detect spirochetes. Penicillin therapy is indicated.
- Episodes of PFAPA are characterised by attacks of unprovoked systemic inflammation with periodic fever. Each episode is followed by a symptom-free interval ranging in duration from weeks to months. Steroids are effective therapy.
- Mouth ulcers are common in Crohn's disease, but rare in ulcerative colitis. Beware that the mouth lesions may precede the intestinal manifestations.
- Oral gels, which are used to treat oral ulcers, may contain salicylate salts. They should not be given to children under 12 years of age as they may cause Reye's syndrome.

- Beware a child with atopic dermatitis who becomes infected with herpes simplex virus resulting in eczema herpeticum. This is the most serious manifestation of herpes virus and may end in death.
- Remember that multiple mouth ulcers may be the first sign of neutropenia or aplastic anaemia.
- Major aphthae, which are difficult to heal, need dental consultation to exclude more serious diseases such as HIV. Other manifestations of HIV include oral candidiasis and periodontitis.
- Beware oral manifestations of child abuse. These may include broken teeth, lip injury or tears to the lingual frenum. Abuse should be thought of if the injury is not compatible with history.

NOTES:

MOUTH BLEEDING

The clinician overview

Mouth bleeding is common in the paediatric population. It is usually mild, not life-threatening, and the cause is found locally. The most common cause is trauma such as cutting the lip or mouth as a result of a fall or running into a solid object. Other causes include inflammation and ulcers. Periodontal diseases (affecting the gingiva, alveolar bone, cementum and periodontal ligament) are other important causes of bleeding. Occasionally, mouth bleeding may be caused by serious underlying systemic disorders such as thrombocytopenia, neutropenia, aplastic anaemia and von Willebrand's disease.

Possible diagnoses

INFANTS
Common
- Trauma (including birth trauma)
- Candidiasis
- Liver cholestasis
- Coagulopathy (e.g. haemophilia)
- Vitamin K deficiency (breastfed infants)

Rare
- Drugs (e.g. methotrexate)

CHILDREN

- Trauma
- Gingivitis
- Thrombocytopenia
- Nosebleed
- Periodontitis

- Viral haemorrhagic fever
- Scurvy
- Child abuse
- Hepatic failure
- Leptospirosis
- Lesch–Nyhan syndrome

Differential diagnosis at a glance

	Trauma	Gingivitis	Thrombocytopenia	Nosebleed	Periodontitis
Purpura on skin	Possible	No	Possible	No	No
Large bleed	Possible	No	Possible	Possible	No
Diagnosis by history	Possible	Possible	Possible	Possible	No
Obvious mouth inflammatory changes	Possible	Yes	No	No	Yes
Associated with pain	Yes	Possible	No	No	Possible

Recommended investigations

***   FBC: to exclude thrombocytopenia, aplastic anaemia.

***   Clotting factors in case of haemorrhagic diathesis (PT, PTT).

***   LFT will confirm liver disease (in cholestasis: high direct bilirubin and alkaline phosphatase).

TOP TIPS

◪ Bleeding from vitamin K deficiency usually occurs within the first 1–7 days of life and rarely as late as 12 weeks. Entirely breastfed infants have a 20 times greater risk of such deficiency than those receiving formula.

◪ Bleeding from the gum or gingivitis is usually due to poor oral hygiene. Prevention of bleeding rests on promoting proper oral hygiene, e.g. regular teeth brushing and use of dental floss.

◪ In case of nosebleed, the child should sit upright with the head tilted forward to ensure that the blood does not run down the throat.

◪ Swallowing of blood from mouth bleeding may cause nausea with subsequent haematemesis.

◪ Beware that blood from nosebleed may flow down the throat and be mistakenly considered as mouth bleed.

◪ Remember that oropharyngeal candidiasis does not bleed unless the white plaque is removed from the underlying tissue, leaving pinpoint haemorrhages. Acute herpetic gingivostomatitis may resemble oral candida.

Red flags

- Mouth bleeding may be the presenting feature of serious underlying diseases such as thrombocytopenia; a clue is when there is no local source of bleeding.
- Beware that mild oral bleeding may go unnoticed because the child continually swallows the blood. Such a child may present with melaena, which may lead to a lot of wrong and unnecessary investigation.
- Child abuse should always be considered as a possible cause if an infant or young child presents with unexplained mouth injury or the injury is not compatible with the history given. In such a case the skin should be examined for bruises; skeletal survey may be necessary.
- Gingivitis may be the presenting symptom of acute non-lymphoblastic leukaemia, thrombocytopenia or neutropenia.

NOTES:

BAD BREATH (HALITOSIS)

The clinician overview

Halitosis is defined as an exhaled air containing more than 75 parts per billion of odour-producing volatile sulphur compounds. This occurs through decomposition of mucous secretion, debris and dental plaque by Gram-negative anaerobes. Halitosis is a symptom caused by various conditions including postnasal drip, dry mouth, dental diseases, sinusitis and gastrointestinal and pulmonary problems. Oral cavity (particularly on the dorsum of the tongue and in areas between teeth) is the most common source of halitosis and is responsible in about 85% of cases. Conditions that predispose to halitosis include a decrease in the flow of saliva, a high amount of protein in the diet, reduced amount of carbohydrates, dental and gum diseases and prolonged intake of antibiotic.

Possible diagnoses

INFANTS
Common
- Mouth inflammation
- Dehydration (e.g. fever)
- Certain foods (e.g. spices)

Rare

CHILDREN

- Poor oral hygiene
- Dehydration (e.g. fever and mouth breathing)
- Pharyngitis/tonsillitis
- Pseudo-halitosis
- Dental diseases

- Gum diseases
- Medications
- Sinusitis
- Bronchiectasis
- Eating certain foods (e.g. garlic, spices)
- Nasal foreign body
- Respiratory, liver and renal diseases

Differential diagnosis at a glance

	Poor oral hygiene	Dehydration	Pharyngitis/ tonsillitis	Pseudo-halitosis	Dental diseases
Dry mouth mucosa	Possible	Yes	Possible	No	Possible
Fever	No	Possible	Yes	No	Possible
Acute onset	No	Possible	Yes	No	Possible
Normal smell	Possible	Possible	Possible	Yes	Possible
Red, inflamed mouth mucosa	No	Possible	Yes	No	Possible

Recommended investigations

No investigations are needed in the vast majority of cases.

TOP TIPS

- ☑ A child presenting with halitosis should be examined by smelling their breath from a distance of 10–15 cm. The odour is scored on a five-point scale. The tongue's odour is measured by scraping the back of the tongue with a plastic spoon and evaluating the smell on the spoon.
- ☑ Beware of any medications taken that cause dry mouth and possible halitosis. These include antihistamine, antidepressant, bronchodilators and anticholinergics.
- ☑ A Halimeter is a useful device to confirm halitosis; the measurement involves a flexible straw being inserted into the mouth or nostril while the patient holds their breath. The measurement is in parts per billion and any measurement more than 75 parts per billion is diagnostic.
- ☑ Beware that the coating on the tongue is often the cause of halitosis. Gentle, daily cleaning of the dorsum of the tongue and mouth rinsing are important. If xerostomia exists, plenty of sugar-free fluids may stimulate the salivary flow.
- ☑ Remember that fever is the most common cause of dry mouth because of increased insensible perspiration. Extra cups of fluids are beneficial for both the fever and the halitosis.
- ☑ Pseudo-halitosis is common and occurs when halitosis actually does not exist but parents (and sometimes children themselves) perceive it as such. Reassurance is all that is needed.
- ☑ If a Halimeter is used to diagnosis halitosis, beware the device is specific for hydrogen sulphide gas, not for methylmercaptan gas, which is also odour producing.

Red flags

- ☑ Beware that halitosis may be a clue to some serious underlying cause such as bronchiectasis or nasal foreign body.

NOTES:

Skin

Pallor and anaemia

Purpura (petechiae and ecchymosis)

Itching (pruritus)

Macules and patches

Papules and plaques

Blisters (vesicles and bullae)

Pustules

Nodules and tumours

Hyper- and hypopigmented lesions

Cyanosis

Telangiectasia

Excessive sweating (hyperhidrosis)

PALLOR AND ANAEMIA

The clinician overview

Normal skin colour is mostly determined by a combination of the child's constitutional degree of melanin content of the skin resulting from hereditary and racial backgrounds. Pallor, reduced or loss of the skin or mucous membrane colour, can be caused by a variety of conditions including normal complexion, lack of exposure to sunlight, anaemia, emotional stress, shock or chronic disease. In neonates, high Hb and RBCs are due to active erythropoiesis in response to low arterial oxygen saturation (AOS) during fetal life. This erythropoiesis ceases abruptly with the rise of AOS at birth. Low erythropoiesis continues for 6–10 weeks causing a decline in Hb to 9–11 g/dL in full-term and 7–9 g/dL in premature infants. This low Hb is the best stimulus for erythropoiesis and should not be suppressed by blood transfusion. Anaemia is defined as an Hb level of less than 11 g/dL. This section will discuss anaemia but a detailed account of the subject is beyond the scope of this book.

Possible diagnoses

INFANTS
Common
- Feto-fetal transfusion
- Blood loss
- Haemolytic anaemia
- Infection
- Physiological anaemia

Rare
- DIC
- Osteopetrosis
- Red cell aplasia (Diamond-Blackfan)
- Hereditary elliptocytosis
- Hereditary stomatocytosis

CHILDREN

- Iron deficiency anaemia (IDA)
- Thalasaemia
- Chronic disease (infection, inflammation, tumour)
- Haemolytic anaemia (e.g. spherocytosis)
- Haemoglobinopathy (e.g. sickle-cell anaemia)

- Lead poisoning
- Drugs (e.g. chemotherapy, aspirin)
- Haemolytic uraemic syndrome
- Autoimmune haemolytic anaemia
- Haemolytic anaemia due to enzymatic defects
- Inflammatory bowel disease (e.g. Crohn's disease (CD))

☑ Hypothyroidism
☑ Storage diseases
☑ Megaloblastic anaemia (folic acid and
  vitamin B_{12} deficiency)
☑ Paroxysmal nocturnal haemoglobulinuria

Differential diagnosis at a glance

	IDA	Thalasaemia	Chronic disease	Haemolytic anaemia	Haemoglobinopathy
Splenomegaly	Possible	Yes	Possible	Yes	Yes
Reticulocytosis	No	Yes	No	Yes	Yes
Low ferritin	Yes	No	Possible	No	No
↓ MCV, MCH	Yes	Yes	Possible	No	No
Hyperbilirubinaemia	No	Yes	Possible	Yes	Yes

Recommended investigations

*** FBC: Hb < 11 g/dL indicates anaemia, low MCV (< 70 fL) and MCH (< 26 pg) suggests microcytic, hypochromic anaemia. Normal WBC and platelets exclude pathologies such as aplastic anaemia.

*** Serum ferritin low in IDA.

*** LFT: hyperbilirubinaemia: suggestive of acute or chronic haemolysis.

*** Reticulocyte count high in haemolytic anaemia, and response to iron treatment.

*** Lead blood level will confirm lead-induced anaemia.

*** Vitamin B_{12} and folate (MCV > 90) to exclude common causes of megaloblastic anaemia.

*** Hb-electrophoresis: HbS in sickle-cell anaemia; high level of HbF to confirm thalasaemia.

** Bone marrow examination is required to exclude other disorders, such as aplastic anaemia.

TOP TIPS

☑ Anaemia of prematurity is very common, and is usually normocytic and normochromic and does not respond to iron therapy. Healthy infants will self-correct provided iron is available.

☑ Blood transfusion is given if the neonate is symptomatic (apnoea, poor weight gain, feeding problems) or if the Hb is < 6.5 g/dL.

☑ Iron supplement should be given to all premature infants until the first year of life.

☑ Pallor is of no great significance unless accompanied by palled lip, mouth, conjunctive and fingernails. If these sites are pale, Hb needs to be checked to exclude anaemia.

☑ Mild anaemia is usually asymptomatic; pallor and clinical symptoms first occur when the Hb falls below 7–8 g/dL.

- By far the most common cause of anaemia is nutritional iron deficiency, which can be easily diagnosed by low Hb, MCV, MCH and ferritin level.
- It can be difficult to exclude thalasaemia from IDA; both have low MCV and MCH. Ferritin can differentiate (normal or high in thalasaemia). Remember that IDA can coexist with thalasaemia; therefore $HbA_2 > 3.4\%$ is diagnostic of thalasaemia trait.
- Treatment with oral iron should be given to all children with Hb < 11 g/dL for 4–6 weeks. Hb needs to be checked to ensure recovery from the anaemia.
- Hb check should be considered in any child with prolonged feeding or dietary problems.
- In districts or localities with a high rate of socio-economic deprivation, IDA is very common.
- IDA may exert an impact on a child's development. School-age children with IDA will have impaired concentration and activity that affects learning.
- Resist the temptation of the parents to add tonics, vitamins or trace metals to iron therapy. These have no scientific value.

Red flags

- Beware that rapid correction of anaemia by transfusion in neonates can be dangerous because of the load impact on circulation and heart. Transfuse slowly small amounts of packed RBCs.
- Ignoring the need to investigate anaemia (even when mild) is a mistake; its presence may indicate a serious underlying disorder.
- Beware that children with CD may present with anaemia alone; ask whether there have been abdominal pain and weight loss; these are the main clinical presentations of CD.
- Iron preparations are an important cause of accidental overdose. Ensure that the parents are keeping the medicine away from children. Parents should also be told about common side effects of iron therapy.

NOTES:

PURPURA (PETECHIAE AND ECCHYMOSIS)

The clinician overview

The normal haemostatic mechanisms are complex but primarily are based on vascular response (vasoconstriction and retraction of blood vessels), decrease in blood flow to the affected area, platelet clot formation and activation of coagulation factors to form fibrin to stabilise the clot. Purpura is due to vasculopathy, thrombocytopathy, coagulopathy or a combination of these mechanisms. It indicates extravasation of blood into the skin or mucosal membranes. Lesions are not raised. Purpura may represent a benign condition or a serious underlying disorder such as meningococcal septicaemia (MCS). Depending on their size, lesions are either petechiae (pinpoint haemorrhages of < 1 cm, usually < 2 mm, in diameter) or ecchymoses (> 1 cm in diameter). In contrast to exanthem and telangiectasia, purpura does not blanch on pressure. In neonates, petechiae are commonly observed on the presenting part during delivery, particularly if the delivery was traumatic. In late infancy and toddlers, bruises frequently occur over bony prominences such as shins, knees and forehead.

Possible diagnoses

INFANTS

Common

- Infection (intrauterine or acquired)
- Hypoxia (disseminated intravascular coagulation (DIC))
- Drugs
- Vitamin K deficiency
- Thrombocytopenia

Rare

- Child abuse
- Thrombocytopenia, absent radius (TAR)
- Kasabach–Merritt syndrome (thrombocytopenia with haemangioma)
- Wiskott–Aldrich syndrome
- Histiocytosis

CHILDREN

- Henoch–Schölein purpura
- Idiopathic thrombocytopenic purpura (ITP)
- Drugs
- Infection (e.g. MCS)
- Physical abuse/trauma

- Bone marrow infiltration/failure (e.g. leukaemia)
- Vascular purpuras (e.g. von Willebrand's disease)
- Hereditary coagulation defects (haemophilia A and B)
- Ehlers–Danlos syndrome
- Liver disease

- Malabsorption
- Haemolytic-uraemic syndrome (HUS)
- Other causes of thrombocytopenia (e.g. postviral infection)
- Scurvy
- Wiskott–Aldrich syndrome
- Post-transfusion purpura

Differential diagnosis at a glance

	HSP	ITP	Drugs	Infection	Physical abuse/ trauma
Petechial	Possible	Yes	Possible	Yes	Possible
Low platelets	No	Yes	Possible	Possible	No
Fever	Possible	No	No	Yes	No
Ill-looking	No	No	No	Yes	No
Preceded URTI	Possible	Possible	No	Possible	No

Recommended investigations

*** Urine to screen for renal involvement in HSP.

*** FBC: to confirm isolated thrombocytopenia; or reduction of all cell lines in cases of marrow infiltration or aplastic anaemia. Blasts suggests leukaemia; leukocytosis in bacterial infection.

*** BC, U&E, calcium, BG, and fibrin degradation products (FDP) with suspected septicaemia.

*** Cerebrospinal fluid in cases of MCD.

*** LFT and U&E for underlying renal and liver disease.

*** Coagulation screen: bleeding and clotting time, PTT (screen for factor VIII; haemophilia) and PT (for factors VII, V, X), clotting factors, such as VIII, IX if PT is abnormal.

*** FDP for DIC.

*** Bone marrow examination indicated if the cause is not obvious (e.g. aleukaemic leukaemia).

TOP TIPS

▪ In a neonate with petechiae, management starts by taking mother's previous medical history for possible ITP, systemic lupus erythematosus, drugs, and infections during pregnancy.

▪ In purpura, careful history and thorough examination are more important than extensive tests.

▪ Baseline tests for most purpuras should include FBC, peripheral blood smear, PT and PTT. Additional tests should be performed when indicated by the history, physical examination and the baseline screening tests.

▪ Distribution of the purpura can offer important clues to the diagnosis: in MCS, lesions are often on the neck and chest; in HSP, the lesions are predominately on the shins, feet and buttocks; in ITP, there is bruising and bleeding from the gums and mucous membrane.

▪ Kasabach–Merritt syndrome is characterised by vascular lesion (haemangioma), thrombocytopenia and chronic consumption coagulopathy. Platelets are consumed and destroyed within the haemangioma.

▪ Remember that infants up to the age of 3–4 months have physiological prolongation of PTT, and that abnormal PT and PTT only occur when coagulation factor levels are < 40%.

▪ Be familiar with multiple bruises of varying ages on the lower legs of young children; these are common and of no significance. Some petechial lesions seen on the face and neck can follow severe coughing or vomiting. These may be mistaken as a sign of septicaemia.

▪ Any acutely ill child with purpura (caused, for example, by MCS) should receive immediate management, including antibiotics, on admission to the emergency department.

▪ Whenever there are unexplained bruises, non-accidental injury (NAI) should always be suspected. Lesions are suspected when they are found in areas of the body not normally subjected to injury (trunk, buttocks and cheeks). Additional clues to NAI should be sought: inflicted cigarette burns, retinal haemorrhages, intra-oral injury and skeletal examination. Radiological skeletal survey may be indicated.

▪ Any purpura with pallor is likely to be serious: bone marrow disease or HUS could be the cause. Admit and investigate.

NOTES:

ITCHING (PRURITUS)

The clinician overview

Pruritus, a sensation to instinctively desire to relieve by scratching, is either generalised or localised. In contrast to adults, generalised pruritis due to systemic diseases (e.g. liver, diabetes mellitus (DM), renal failure) is rare compared with localised pruritus in children. Pruritus of the perianal area (e.g. nappy rash, atopic dermatitis, threadworms, tight and warm clothing), vulva (non-specific vulvovaginitis) and hair areas (pediculosis, scabies) are the usual sites of localised pruritus. The most common causes of generalised pruritus are dry skin, which is very often inherited as an autosomal dominant, allergic rash such as urticaria, atopic dermatitis (AD) or skin infection.

(Itchy scalp will not be discussed in this section; instead, *see* Hair and nails chapter.)

Possible diagnoses

INFANTS
Common
- ☑ AD
- ☑ Cholestasis
- ☑ Too-warm environment
- ☑ Scabies/pediculosis
- ☑ Varicella

Rare
- ☑ Allergic rash (e.g. urticaria)
- ☑ Drugs

CHILDREN

- ☑ AD
- ☑ Food allergy
- ☑ Dry skin
- ☑ Parasites (scabies and pediculosis, insects, worms)
- ☑ Allergic rash (e.g. urticaria)

- ☑ Varicella
- ☑ Drugs (e.g. chlorpromazine)
- ☑ Chronic renal failure (CRF)
- ☑ Endocrine (DM, hyper- or hypothyroidism)
- ☑ Dermatitis herpetiformis
- ☑ Psychogenic
- ☑ Iron-deficiency anaemia
- ☑ Polycythaemia
- ☑ Lichen planus

- Liver disease (obstructive jaundice)
- Pregnancy
- Sea bather's eruption
- Certain malignancy (e.g. Hodgkin's lymphoma)
- Serum sickness

Differential diagnosis at a glance

	AD	Food allergy	Dry skin	Parasites	Allergic rash
Generalised	No	Yes	Yes	No	Yes
Mainly on flexures	Yes	No	No	No	No
Worse at night	Yes	No	Possible	Possible	No
Cause obvious on skin	Yes	No	Yes	Possible	Yes
+ family history	Yes	Possible	Yes	Possible	No

Recommended investigations

**   Urinalysis: dipstick for glycosuria to suggest DM.

***   FBC will confirm anaemia in iron-deficiency anaemia, eosinophilia in allergic conditions and worm infestation; high WBC may suggest leukaemia.

***   U&E will diagnose CRF.

***   LFT: hyperbilirubinaemia in jaundiced patients.

***   TFT to confirm hypothyroidism or hyperthyroidism.

***   Identification of scabies requires scrapings taken from a scabies burrow, then mixed with clear solution (even water) and examined microscopically.

TOP TIPS

- The vast majority of conditions causing pruritus are obvious and the diagnosis is clinical.
- Although localised itching predominates in children, in infancy such itching usually presents as restlessness and discomfort with excessive crying, particularly at night.
- In cases of AD, there is no cure or short cut to the long-term management. Treatment is aimed at relieving the symptoms, including the itching.
- Pruritus is always present in AD; if absent, the diagnosis is incorrect.
- Sea bather's eruption, primarily described in the waters of Florida and the Caribbean, consists of inflammatory papules that develop in about 12 hours of bathing in salt water.
- Remember that seborrhoeic dermatitis (SD) is often difficult to differentiate from AD: pruritus is always present in AD, in contrast to SD.

◪ Any perianal pruritus at night should alert the clinician to the presence of worms. Inspection of the area by parents while the child is asleep often confirms the diagnosis.

Red flags

◪ Any skin dermatosis with intense pruritus, particularly when the child is in bed, should alert the clinician to the presence of scabies.
◪ Beware that scratching due to pruritus results in redness, excoriated papules and infection of the skin. Treatment of these secondary effects is unsuccessful unless the underlying cause (e.g. dry skin) is treated.
◪ Beware that generalised pruritus could be the presenting symptom of obstructive jaundice before the jaundice appears (e.g. primary biliary cirrhosis, drug-induced); the same is true in CRF.

NOTES:

MACULES AND PATCHES

The clinician overview

Macule, known in lay language as dot, is a circumscribed, flat area of change in skin colour that is < 1 cm in diameter. It can be either hyperpigmented (e.g. freckles) or hypopigmented (vitiligo). Patch is a larger area of change in skin colour that is > 1 cm in diameter. The appearance of macules or patches does not commonly remain static, and acute eruptions can change rapidly to become elevated (maculopapular) or blistering (maculovesicular). Therefore, initial rashes that may not be diagnosed on day one may be diagnosed on the following day when the rash reaches its ultimate evolution of appearance before the usual healing.

Possible diagnoses

INFANTS
Common

- Mongolian spots
- Cutis marmorata
- Salmon patch
- Congenital melanocytic naevus
- Nappy rash

Rare

- Port wine stains
- Tuberous sclerosis (hypopigmented ash leaf)
- Cellulitis
- Omphalitis

CHILDREN

- Freckles
- Bruises
- Viral exanthem (specific, e.g. measles, or non-specific)
- Café-au-lait spots (e.g. neurofibromatosis type 1)
- Drug eruption

- Port wine stains
- Lentigo
- Albinism
- Tuberous sclerosis (TS) (or ash leaf spots)
- Post-inflammatory depigmentation
- Vitiligo
- Intertrigo
- Pityriasis (alba, rubra pilaris)
- Post-inflammatory hyper- or hypopigmentation
- Tinea versicolour
- Erythema migrans (Lyme disease)

- Rheumatic diseases (salmon-pink in rheumatoid arthritis)
- Morphea (localised scleroderma)
- Erysipelas

Differential diagnosis at a glance

	Freckles	Bruises	Viral exanthem	Café-au-lait spots	Drug eruption
Fever	No	No	Yes	No	Possible
Blanch on pressure	No	No	Yes	No	Possible
Present at birth	No	Possible	No	Yes	No
Worse by sunlight	Yes	No	No	No	Possible
Inherited	Yes	No	No	Yes	No

Recommended investigations

Usually, in the vast majority of lesions, no special investigations are required as the diagnosis is mostly clinical. In some specific cases the following points are useful.

***   Wood's light to enhance visualisation of hypopigmented lesions of ash leaf in TS.

**   Skin scrapings may be required for a suspected case of tinea versicolour.

**   Acute and post-convalescent serum samples are occasionally required to confirm rubella.

***   A CT scan to confirm calcification in Sturge–Weber syndrome or tuberous sclerosis.

TOP TIPS

- Salmon patch is by far the most common vascular lesion in neonates, with a midline or symmetrical pink maculae over both eyelids.
- Mongolian spots are present at birth in over 80% of Black and Asian children and in 5%–10% of White infants. They may be solitary over the sacral area but can be multiple over the legs and shoulders.
- Because a specific dermatological diagnosis often cannot be made, classification of child's skin disease into groups, e.g. as maculopapular and vesiculobullous, is a good start.
- A child's skin is more reactive than an adult's, e.g. more susceptible to develop warts, vesicles or exanthem following a viral infection.
- For café-au-lait spots, the hallmark of neurofibromatosis, there should be six or more spots over 0.5 cm in diameter in pre-pubertal individuals and over 1.5 cm in diameter (patch) in post-pubertal individuals before the diagnosis can be made.
- Pityriasis versicolour can be hypopigmented (which needs to be differentiated from vitiligo if they appear around the lips) and hyperpigmented.

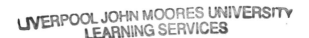

- Mongolian spots (bluish, present at birth) should not be confused with bruises.
- Freckles around the mouth should be differentiated from Peutz–Jeghers syndrome.
- Congenital melanocytic naevus occurs in 1% of all neonates; melanomas rarely develop on these naevi, spontaneous regression may occur.
- One to two lesions of café-au-lait 1–3 cm in length occur in about 20% of all healthy children; they have nothing to do with neurofibromatosis.

- Port wine stain is always present at birth. When it is localised to the trigeminal area of the face, the diagnosis is Sturge–Weber syndrome. Beware of glaucoma and seizure as a complication. CT scan of the head is likely to show calcification.
- Any infant with erythema that surrounds the umbilicus should be regarded as having omphalitis, and the infant should be evaluated for sepsis and parenteral antibiotic treatment.
- Omphalitis, an erythema with purulent umbilical discharge, is a serious neonatal infection, which may spread to adjacent tissue causing peritonitis, hepatic vein thrombosis and hepatic abscess. Immediate septic workup and parenteral antibiotics are required.
- Don't mistake pityriasis alba, which consists of areas of hypopigmentation, with vitiligo. The borders of the lesions of pityriasis, in contrast to vitiligo, are not sharply demarcated. Children with pityriasis can be reassured, along with their parents, that complete restoration of normal skin colour will occur; this is not so with vitiligo.
- Although patches of bruises over the shins are almost universal in toddlers due to frequent falls, bruises on the arms, back, abdomen, thighs and genitalia may be caused by physical child abuse.

NOTES:

PAPULES AND PLAQUES

The clinician overview

A papule, little bump in lay language, is a small (< 1 cm) elevated lesion that is palpable above the skin's surface. A plaque is a raised lesion with its surface area greater than the elevation. Plaques vary in size from 1 cm to a huge size covering part of the body. Plaques can arise directly from the skin or through a coalescence of papules. Some eruptions have a combination of papules and plaques (papulosquamous eruption).

Possible diagnoses

INFANTS
Common
- ☑ Erythema toxicum neonatorum
- ☑ Milia
- ☑ Neonatal acne
- ☑ Scabies
- ☑ Contact dermatitis

Rare
- ☑ Histiocytosis syndrome (histiocytosis X)
- ☑ Mastocytosis

CHILDREN
Common
- ☑ Acne
- ☑ Atopic dermatitis
- ☑ Warts
- ☑ Molluscum contagiosum
- ☑ Insect bite

- ☑ Scabies
- ☑ Gottron's papule (in dermatomyositis)
- ☑ Contact dermatitis
- ☑ Discoid lupus erythematosus
- ☑ Psoriasis (papules in guttate form, otherwise plaques)
- ☑ Papular urticaria
- ☑ Pityriasis rosea
- ☑ Lichen planus
- ☑ Histiocytosis syndrome (histiocytosis X)
- ☑ Fungal infection
- ☑ Granuloma annulare
- ☑ Fabry's disease
- ☑ Cat-scratch fever

Differential diagnosis at a glance

	Acne	Atopic dermatitis	Warts	Molluscum contagiosum	Insect bite
Severe itching	No	Yes	No	No	Possible
Associated pain	No	No	No	No	Yes
Exposed area	Yes	No	Yes	No	Yes
Adolescent age	Yes	No	No	Yes	No
Umbilicated centre	No	No	No	Yes	No

Recommended investigations

Usually, in the vast majority of lesions, no special investigations are required as the diagnosis is mostly clinical. In some specific cases the following points are useful.

***   Scraping of scabies burrow to be mixed with a clear solution (e.g. water) and examined microscopically.

**   Skin biopsy to confirm histiocytosis.

TOP TIPS

- Milia, white papules of retention cysts and 1–2 mm in size, are very common in neonates (about 50%); they are seen on the nose and disappear quickly. A pearly papule 1–2 mm on the midline of the palate, Epstein pearl, is a milium, which also disappears later on.
- Psoriasis may present as guttates, which are silvery scaly papules usually seen on the trunk and often following streptococcal throat infection. About one-quarter of all psoriasis sufferers develop their disease in childhood. Knees, elbows, buttocks and nails are common sites.
- Lichen planus is not that uncommon in children. Lesions are polygonal, flat-topped papules, 2–6 mm in diameter. Diagnosis can often be confirmed by white papules on the buccal mucosa.
- Scabies, which is characterised by papules, usually excoriated, often presents as dermatitis and is often mistaken as atopic dermatitis. The presence of burrows from which parasites can be found can separate the two conditions.

- ☑ Mastocytosis, accumulation of mast cells in the skin, can either present as disseminated plaques or in solitary, nodular form (mastocytoma). Beware that systemic signs of mastocytosis (e.g. syncope, hypotension and flushing) may precede the development of skin lesions.
- ☑ Erythema toxicum neonatorum, seen in about half of healthy newborns, is often mistaken as staphylococcal pustules. The well-appearing child and the asymptomatic rash exclude any infection.
- ☑ Histiocytosis (previously known as histiocytosis X), can be mistaken as the more common seborrhoeic dermatitis if it affects the scalp, or atopic dermatitis if it infiltrates the trunk. Histiocytosis may present with immunodeficiency and progressive CNS involvement.

NOTES:

BLISTERS (VESICLES AND BULLAE)

The clinician overview

Blister is the lay terminology for both vesicle and bulla. While a vesicle is a fluid-filled raised cavity that is < 1 cm in diameter, a bulla is > 1 cm in diameter. Vesicles may occur on the mucosa of the mouth; it is, however, unusual to see them intact because there is so much friction and trauma from moving the tongue and eating. Vesiculobullous eruptions indicate that blisters are the primary lesions. Such eruptions can be caused by infection such as varicella, bullous impetigo, herpes simplex, hereditary blistering disorders such as epidermolysis bullosa, external factors such as sunburn and contact dermatitis, or by immune-mediated cutaneous diseases such as dermatitis herpetiformis, bullous pemphigoid and pemphigus.

Possible diagnoses

INFANTS
Common
- Erythema toxicum neonatorum
- Staphylococcal infection
- Herpes simplex virus
- Herpetic gingivostomatitis
- Sucking blisters

Rare
- Epidermolysis bullosa
- Epidermolytic hyperkeratosis
- Incontinentia pigmenti (first phase of the disease)
- Toxic epidermal necrolysis (Lyell's syndrome)
- Neonatal pemphigus vulgaris
- Bullous mastocytosis
- Congenital syphilis
- Dermatitis herpetiformis
- Staphylococcal scalded skin syndrome
- Bullous impetigo
- Pemphigus vulgaris

CHILDREN
- Varicella (chickenpox)
- Herpes simplex
- Herpes zoster
- Erythema multiforme (EM)
- Bullous impetigo

- Eczema herpeticum
- Porphyria
- Stevens–Johnson syndrome
- Drug allergy (bullous drug eruption)
- Naproxen-induced pseudoporphyria
- Hand-foot-mouth disease

☑ Contact dermatitis
☑ Linear IgA dermatosis

Differential diagnosis at a glance

	Varicella	Herpes simplex	Herpes zoster	EM	Bullous impetigo
Vesicles	Yes	Yes	Yes	Possible	Possible
Bullae	No	No	No	Yes	Yes
Mucosal involvement	Yes	Possible	No	Yes	No
Fever	Possible	Possible	Possible	Possible	No
Unilateral	No	No	Yes	No	No

Recommended investigations

**   Blood to screen for autoimmune diseases (such as ANA).

***   Screening tests for Crohn's disease, serum IgA-endomysial antibodies for cases of dermatitis herpetiformis.

**   Culture of swabs from the lesions of bullous impetigo may help identify the infecting bacteria.

**   Biopsy of the lesions is sometimes indicated for diagnostic purposes for such immune-mediated blistering diseases as pemphigus or dermatitis herpetiformis

TOP TIPS

☑ Note that the vesicles that are situated superficially are flaccid and rupture easily (e.g. bullous impetigo) whereas those arising from deeper layers are more tense.

☑ The diagnosis of erythema multiforme is based on target lesions with an erythematous outer border, an inner pale ring and a dark dusky centre.

☑ Hand-foot-mouth disease is a benign, common infection caused by A16 strain of coxsakievirus, and usually arises first on the soft palate and tongue followed by cutaneous lesions 1–2 days later.

☑ Nikolsky's sign (gentle rubbing produces similar skin lesions) is a useful test. This is positive in conditions like staphylococcal scalded skin syndrome, toxic epidermal necrolysis and pemphigus.

☑ Bullae at birth may be the first manifestation of epidermolysis bullosa. Bullae caused by staphylococci are usually not present at birth and the bullae fluid appears infected in contrast to the clear uninfected fluid in epidermolysis bullosa.

☑ Beware that EM may affect the oral mucosa (in 25% of cases), typically affects the lip border and buccal mucosa but sparing the gingiva. The lesions are benign and disappear within 2 weeks.

◪ In contrast to adults, childhood herpes zoster is not commonly associated with localised pain or postherpetic neuralgia. Immunocompromised children may have a severe zoster that is similar to that in adults.

Red flags

◪ Herpes zoster (shingles) is relatively benign, except when it affects the ophthalmic division, which can affect the vision.
◪ Naproxen, a non-steroidal anti-inflammatory drug used as an inflammatory agent in rheumatic diseases, may cause a severe eruption characterised by erythema, vesicles or bullae and shallow atrophic scars after sun exposure (toxic epidermal necrolysis and pseudoporphyria).
◪ Don't attempt incising or puncturing bullae as this may induce infection.
◪ Eczema herpeticum is a serious infection caused by herpes simplex virus that is invading eczematous lesions. It can lead to death through dissemination of the virus to the brain and other organs or from secondary staphylococcal or streptococcal infection.
◪ Herpes simplex and varicella can become disseminated and life-threatening in immunocompromised patients. Admit and give IV acyclovir, possibly with other medications.

NOTES:

PUSTULES

The clinician overview

A pustule is a superficial, elevated lesion containing pus. It may primarily result from a bacterial infection, usually staphylococcal, or when the content of a vesicle or bulla becomes secondarily infected. Pustules are similar to vesicles, but the fluid they contain is a purulent exudate resulting from accumulation of leukocytes, microorganisms and cellular debris. It may occur either as a primary (e.g. bullous impetigo) or secondary infection (e.g. infected atopic dermatitis). When pustules arise at the opening of hair follicles, the condition is termed folliculitis. Not all pustules have infectious contents, e.g. the contents of transient neonatal pustulosis are sterile without microorganisms if cultured.

Possible diagnoses

INFANTS
Common
- Erythema toxicum neonatorum (ETN)
- Staphylococcal infection
- Transient neonatal pustulosis
- Bullous impetigo
- Neonatal acne

Rare
- Congenital varicella
- Eosinophilic pustular folliculitis
- Infantile acropustulosis
- Staphylococcal pustulosis

CHILDREN
- Infected atopic dermatitis (AD)
- Impetigo
- Acne
- Varicella
- Staphylococcal skin infection (e.g. furuncle, carbuncle)

- Infected pediculosis
- Eosinophilic pustular folliculitis
- Infantile acropustulosis
- Staphylococcal pustulosis

Differential diagnosis at a glance

	Infected AD	Impetigo	Acne	Varicella	Staphylococcal skin infection
Presence of comedones	No	No	Yes	No	No
Mucosal involvement	No	No	No	Yes	No
Fever	Possible	No	No	Yes	Possible
Severe pruritus	Yes	Possible	Possible	Yes	Possible
Perioral involvement	No	Yes	No	Possible	Possible

Recommended investigations

In the vast majority of lesions, no special investigations are required as the diagnosis is mostly clinical. In some cases swab from any pus or open infected lesion to confirm the organism.

TOP TIPS

◪ Not all pustules are representing infection, some fluids inside are sterile, e.g. transient neonatal pustular melanosis, which is a benign, self-limited dermatosis of unknown aetiology and requires no treatment.

◪ Varicella lesions evolve from erythematous macules to form papules. Over the next 2 days there will be pustules that rupture to form crusts. Lesions are typically polymorphic.

◪ Papules and pustules around the mouth are often due to staphylococcal or streptococcal infection; treat with an antibiotic, not a topical steroid.

◪ Beware that lesions of ETN are often pustules that have to be differentiated from similar-appearing staphylococcal infection. A child with ETN is well and asymptomatic.

Red flags

◪ It is important to differentiate neonatal varicella (NV) from congenital varicella syndrome (CVS). CVS occurs when pregnant women contract varicella at 6–20 weeks of gestation; about 25% of neonates may develop varicella embryopathy (such as limb interruption, eye involvement, cicatrical scarring). NV occurs if the fetus is born within a week of maternal varicella resulting in a severe form of varicella because of lack of transplacental antibody to the virus.

◪ Herpes simplex or zoster in an immunocompromised child indicates serious infection; urgent management and appropriate treatment (with acyclovir) are required.

☑ Recurrent staphylococcal infections require investigations as this may suggest a systemic disease or immunosuppression.

NOTES:

NODULES AND TUMOURS

The clinician overview

Nodule is a palpable, solid lesion of more than 0.5–1.0 mm in diameter. Examples are small fibroma, erythema nodosum and skin tumour. Larger nodules (> 20 mm) are classified as tumour, benign or malignant. Nodules and tumour are circumscribed, elevated lesions that are larger than papules and that arise from deeper structure, thus displaying elevation as well as depth. Tumour can arise from deeper as well as superficial structures such as the dermis or the epidermis.

Possible diagnoses

INFANTS
Common
- Warts
- Subcutaneous fat necrosis
- Dermoid cyst
- Haemangioma
- Infantile digital fibroma

Rare
- Mastocytoma
- Neonatal lupus erythematosus
- Metastatic neuroblastoma
- Reticulohistiocytosis (Hashimoto–Pritzker disease)

CHILDREN

- Fibroma (or lipoma)
- Dermoid cyst
- Nodulocystic acne
- Erythema nodosum
- Haemangioma

- Keloid
- Discoid lupus erythematosus
- Panniculitis
- Granular cell tumour, basal cell carcinoma
- Cystic hygroma
- Juvenile xanthogranuloma
- Hidradenitis
- Rheumatoid nodule
- Malignant melanoma
- Rheumatoid nodules
- Xanthoma
- Malignant melanoma
- Sarcoidosis
- Juvenile xanthogranuloma
- Nevus (such as Spitz's or sebaceous nevus)

Differential diagnosis at a glance

	Fibroma	Dermoid cyst	Nodulocystic acne	Erythema nodosum	Haemangioma
Present in neonate	Possible	Yes	No	No	Yes
Skin-coloured	Yes	Yes	No	No	No
Presence of comedones	No	No	Yes	No	No
Tenderness	No	No	Possible	Yes	No
Regress spontaneously	Possible	No	Yes	Yes	Yes

Recommended investigations

Usually, in the vast majority of lesions, no special investigations are required as the diagnosis is mostly clinical. In some specific cases the following points are useful.

** FBC: may reveal anaemia in case of chronic inflammatory diseases.

** Rheumatoid factor: positive with the presence of rheumatoid nodules.

** Kveim test: is a useful test in case of sarcoidosis.

** Biopsy for obscure nodular lesion.

TOP TIPS

☑ It is important to describe the colour, surface shape, outline, elevation, depth, mobility and degree of firmness in every case with nodules or tumours.

☑ Subcutaneous fat necrosis is a self-resolving and benign condition seen on areas of pressure (cheeks, buttocks, thighs) in healthy newborns.

☑ Haemangiomas are found in about 10% of all children. They are usually not present at birth but appear in the first few weeks of life, enlarge during early infancy and regress at 4–6 years of age.

☑ Haemangiomas occur in a number of syndromes, including PHACE syndrome, which is associated with segmental facial haemangioma with posterior malformation of the brain and arterial anomalies such as coarctation of the aorta.

☑ Erythema nodosum is an important skin lesion characterised by subcutaneous, tender nodules on the lower legs, pretibial. The underlying cause may be streptococcal infection, TB, sarcoidosis or inflammatory bowel diseases.

☑ Note that mastocytoma (accumulation of mast cells in the skin) occurs almost exclusively in infancy as a reddish or orange nodule that is rubbery in consistency.

☑ Keloid, in contrast to a hypertrophic scar, extends its growth beyond the limit of the original scar and does not regress spontaneously. Both result from trauma to the skin, e.g. from surgical procedure.

◪ Infantile digital fibroma (firm skin-coloured or erythematous nodule at the lateral surfaces of the distal phalanges) has to be differentiated from subungual or periungual fibroma, which is related to tuberous sclerosis and tends to occur after puberty.

Red flags

◪ Any unexplained nodule in the skin requires urgent referral to a dermatologist to obtain a diagnosis as soon as possible.
◪ Although basal cell carcinoma is rare in children, it may result from basal cell nevus, radiotherapy for other malignancies or after excessive sun exposure.
◪ Although malignant melanoma is typically an adult tumour, just under 2% can occur during childhood. Attention has to be paid to this potentially fatal disease; irregular or notched borders, bleeding or ulceration and colour changes may all suggest malignant change.
◪ Some nevi look like malignant melanoma; a biopsy may be needed to distinguish the two lesions.

NOTES:

HYPER- AND HYPOPIGMENTED LESIONS

The clinician overview

Pigmentary disorders are a common presentation to general practitioners, paediatricians and dermatologists. In some cases, pigmentation is an external sign of a serious underlying systemic disorder. In general, children who present with multiple or generalised hyperpigmented lesions have a more serious underlying disease than those who present with isolated lesions. Increased pigmentation, caused by deposition of melanin, may be due to hormonal changes, e.g. pregnancy, or increased melanogenesis as in haemochromatosis. It may be generalised or localised, result from defects in melanocyte formation, production, differentiation, migration or distribution. Hypopigmentation or depigmentation indicates a congenital or acquired decrease in melanin production. In some cases, e.g. tuberous sclerosis (TS), hyper-and hypopigmented lesions occur.

Hyperpigmentation

Possible diagnoses

INFANTS
Common
- Carotenaemia
- Café-au-lait
- Junctional nevi
- Post-inflammatory hyperpigmentation
- Other neurocutaneous syndrome (e.g. TS)

Rare
- Giant or small hairy nevus
- Albright's syndrome
- Congenital Addison's disease
- Fanconi's syndrome
- Generalised hereditary lentigines
- Androgen excess

CHILDREN
- Freckles (ephelides)
- Lentigines
- Café-au-lait
- Post-inflammatory hyperpigmentation (PIH)
- Mastocytosis (urticaria pigmentosa, mastocytoma)

- Other neurocutaneous syndrome (e.g. tuberous sclerosis)
- Incontinentia pigmenti
- Peutz–Jeghers syndrome
- LEOPARD syndrome
- LAMB syndrome
- Addison's disease
- Melanoma
- Fanconi's syndrome
- Androgen excess
- Drugs
- Acanthosis nigricans
- Pregnancy

Differential diagnosis at a glance

	Freckles	Lentigines	Café-au-lait	PIH	Mastocytosis
Present at birth	No	Yes	Yes	No	Yes
Sun-exposed area	Yes	No	No	No	No
Previous skin inflammation	No	No	No	Yes	No
+ family history	Yes	Yes	Possible	No	No
Size > 1 cm	No	Yes	Yes	Yes	Yes

Recommended investigations

Usually, in the vast majority of lesions, no special investigations are required as the diagnosis is mostly clinical. In some specific cases the following point is useful.

**   Biopsy for suspected melanoma, with a few millimetres of normal skin surrounding the lesion.

TOP TIPS

▱ Freckles are dark or brown macules, 2–3 mm in diameter with poorly defined margins that occur in sun-exposed areas, particularly the face, upper back, arms and hands.

▱ Lentigines are larger in size than freckles, unrelated to sun exposure and remain permanently. Like freckles, they are benign.

▱ LAMB syndrome is characterised by facial lentigines in addition to atrial myxoma, mucocutaneous myxoma and blue nevi.

▱ LEOPARD syndrome consists of lentigines, in association with ECG abnormalities, ocular hypertelorism, pulmonary stenosis, abnormal genitalia, growth retardation and deafness.

▱ Peutz–Jeghers syndrome consists of hyperpigmented macules, in association with gastrointestinal polyposis.

▱ Mastocytosis is a group of disorders that are characterised by accumulation of mast cells in the skin and other organs. Mastocytoma: a benign cutaneous tumour that occurs exclusively in infancy; urticaria pigmentosa: multiple small salmon-coloured or red cutaneous papules; systemic mastocytosis: mast cell infiltrates in the skin, lymph nodes, liver, spleen, bone, gastrointestinal tract.

▱ Carotenaemia, yellow discolouration of the infant skin due to deposition of the pigment carotene, must be differentiated from jaundice by the presence of a healthy and thriving infant with normal, not jaundiced, sclera. In case of uncertainty, serum bilirubin will differentiate.

▱ A child with multiple pigmented lesions should be considered as having a systemic disease rather than a dermatological problem.

▱ Paediatricians and general practitioners should have a very low threshold for referral to a dermatologist when children present because of parental concern about growth or change in a mole.

▱ Although multiple café-au-lait spots are the hallmark of NF-1, healthy individuals may have few; other diseases may exhibit these lesions, e.g. TS and McCune–Albright syndrome.

▱ Although melanoma is rare in children, excessive exposure to sunlight increases the risk of developing this tumour. Other risk factors include fair skin, atypical moles larger than 5 mm and irregular borders and pigmentation.

▱ Children with Peutz–Jeghers syndrome are at high risk of gastrointestinal malignancy (up to 50% of all cases); close observation is essential.

NOTES:

Hypopigmentation

Possible diagnoses

INFANTS

Common

- Nevus depigmentosus
- Partial albinism (piebaldism)
- Nevus anaemicus

Rare

CHILDREN

- Vitiligo
- Post-inflammatory hypopigmentation
- Pityriasis alba
- Albinism
- Post-varicella depigmentation

- Waardenburg's syndrome
- Chédiak–Higashi syndrome
- Ash leaf spots of tuberous sclerosis
- Infectious hypopigmentation (e.g. tinea versicolour)

Differential diagnosis at a glance

	Vitiligo	Post-inflammatory hypopigmentation	Pityriasis alba	Albinism	Post-varicella depigmentation
Exposed area	No	No	Yes	Yes	Yes
May present at birth	No	No	No	Yes	No
Sharply demarcated	Yes	No	No	No	No
Inherited	Possible	No	No	Yes	No
Mainly on trunk	No	No	No	No	Yes

Recommended investigations

Usually, in the vast majority of lesions, no special investigations are required as the diagnosis is mostly clinical. In some specific cases the following points are useful.

** A skin scrape may be needed to rule out tinea versicolour from the common hypopigmented spots of pityriasis alba.

** Autoantibody screen may be carried out for children with widespread vitiligo.

*** For children with TS, CT scan to diagnose calcification or tumour; ultrasound scan for any renal tumour; echocardiography for rhabdomyoma.

TOP TIPS

▨ Nevus depigmentation is characterised by localised areas of hypopigmentation that are usually present at birth.

▨ About one-half of patients with vitiligo have their lesions during childhood. Antibodies to melanocytes are frequently found suggesting an autoimmune cause. A number of autoimmune diseases occur in the patients and their relatives.

▨ Pityriasis alba, a very common condition characterised by ill-defined hypopigmented spots, 1–2 cm in diameter, on the face, arms and neck.

▨ Nevus anaemicus (an area of localised vasoconstriction) may be mistaken for ash leaf hypopigmentation; the former is blanchable while the latter does not disappear on blanching.

▨ Vitiligo lesions may progress and become universal.

▨ Beware that the lack of protective melanin leads children with albinism to high sun sensitivity, which results in a high incidence of basal and squamous cell carcinoma.

▨ Children with albinism must learn to protect themselves against sun exposure to avoid complications such as skin tumours (basal and squamous cell carcinoma).

▨ In children with widespread albinism, visual impairment is the rule; the more severe the hypopigmentation, the more severe the visual acuity.

NOTES:

CYANOSIS

Cyanosis is caused by the presence of an excess of deoxygenated haemoglobin, which is visible in the skin and mucous membranes (central cyanosis). The great majority of cyanotic children have either pulmonary or cardiac cause. However, clinicians should be aware of cyanosis occurring in healthy normal children; for example, peripheral cyanosis (acrocyanosis) noted in a vast majority of newly born babies (causing Apgar score to be 9 instead of complete 10) and in infants who are unwrapped and cold. Some healthy children may have perioral cyanosis in response to cold with or without shivering, or following a rapid rise of fever. The causes of cardiac and pulmonary cyanosis are large and beyond the scope of this section.

Possible diagnoses

INFANTS

Common

- Acrocyanosis at birth
- Respiratory distress syndrome
- Cyanotic congenital heart disease (CHD)
- Pulmonary hypertension
- Breath-holding attacks

Rare

- Shock and sepsis
- Central hypoventilation
- Methaemoglobinaemia (congenital)
- High Hb (polycythaemia)
- Neuromuscular diseases (e.g. spinal muscular atrophy)

CHILDREN

- Breath holding attacks
- Cardiac (failure, CHD)
- Pulmonary (pneumonia, severe asthma, pneumothorax)
- Fever (onset with shivering)
- Raynaud's phenomenon

- Shock and sepsis (e.g. meningococcal infection)
- Neuromuscular diseases (e.g. muscular dystrophy)
- Methaemoglobinaemia (ingestion of aniline dyes/nitrites)
- Foreign body

Differential diagnosis at a glance

	Breath-holding attacks	Cardiac	Pulmonary	Fever	Raynaud's phenomenon
Transient	Yes	No	Possible	Yes	Yes
Abolished by 100% oxygen	No	No	Yes	No	No
Respiratory distress (e.g. recession, grunting)	No	Possible	Yes	No	No
Low O_2 saturation	No	Yes	Yes	Possible	No
Peripheral	Possible	No	No	Possible	Yes

Recommended investigations

*** FBC to diagnose anaemia and polycythaemia. WBC raised in bacterial infection.

*** Blood gases, with or without breathing 100% oxygen, that results in rapid improvement of the O_2 saturation in pulmonary and central hypoventilation, but not in cardiac diagnosis.

*** Chest X-ray, as the most helpful investigation, can differentiate between pulmonary (e.g. infiltration, pleural effusion, atelectasis, tumour) and cardiac causes (heart enlargement).

** ECG may show ventricular enlargement, arrhythmia or conduction defects.

*** Echocardiography will provide significant help in diagnosis.

*** Lung function tests, including oxygen saturation by oximeter.

TOP TIPS

- ☑ The three main signs of CHD are cyanosis, congestive cardiac failure and the presence of a heart murmur.
- ☑ Most cyanotic CHD will present during the first week of life, usually associated with heart failure cardiac shunt as the cause of the cyanosis, as opposed to a primary pulmonary cause.
- ☑ Hypoxia may occur in the absence of cyanosis (e.g. in anaemia), and cyanosis in the absence of hypoxia (e.g. in polycythaemia).
- ☑ Breathing 100% oxygen will help to differentiate between right-to-left (O_2 saturation remains low) and pulmonary or central hypoventilation.
- ☑ Increased Hb (polycythaemia) is more common in newborns (e.g. following twin-to-twin transfusion, infants of diabetic mothers) than at any age later in childhood.
- ☑ Note that when a child manifests with blue lower extremities and pink upper extremities (differential cyanosis), the child has right-to-left shunt across a ductus arteriosus in the presence of coarctation or interrupted aortic arch.
- ☑ Beware that healthy infants and toddlers may exhibit blue lips when crying vigorously.
- ☑ Mild cyanosis is best detected over the nail beds, lips, tongue and mucous membranes.

■ Methaemoglobinaemia is either congenital, due to autosomal recessive inheritance, or acquired, caused by ingestion of aniline dyes or nitrates. Cyanosis is a predominant feature. Children are otherwise healthy, not in distress and physical examination is normal. Cyanosis is reversed by administration of vitamin C.

Red flags

■ Central hypoventilation is caused by central nervous system diseases such as intracranial haemorrhage or meningitis. The child may present with slow respiration or apnoea.
■ Breath-holding attacks are common in infants and toddlers. After the onset children stop breathing, become blue and may have seizures. In epileptic seizure, children first have a seizure and then become blue.
■ The history and physical examination can always differentiate between cyanotic CHD (persistent cyanosis) and breath-holding attacks (brief and reversible).
■ For any infant with cyanosis suspected of having CHD, referral to a cardiac unit is essential. Before transporting the baby, ensure that a prostaglandin infusion to prevent closure of the ductus arteriosus has been set up.
■ A child who becomes suddenly breathless, choking with or without cyanosis, should be suspected of inhaling a foreign body. Every clinician should be knowledgeable in the management of eliminating it.
■ Pneumothorax could well be the cause of an asthmatic child who becomes suddenly cyanosed and breathless.

NOTES:

TELANGIECTASIA

The clinician overview

Telangiectasia indicates permanently dilated superficial blood vessels in the skin or mucous membranes. One or two telangiectases on the face are very common and trivial in children; they are highly characteristic in their vascular centres, from which radiate fine vessels that give the appearance of a spider's web. Pressure on the central vessel will blanch the lesion. The face and the dorsa of the hands are common sites. The presence of telangiectasia may suggest serious systemic disease such as ataxia telangiectasia, Raynaud's phenomenon (RP) caused by systemic scleroderma and hereditary haemorrhagic telangiectasia (Osler–Weber–Rendu disease).

Possible diagnoses

INFANTS
Common

CHILDREN

- Spider angioma
- Pregnancy/oestrogen treatment
- Liver disease
- Connective tissue diseases (including RP, CREST syndrome)
- Hereditary haemorrhagic telangiectasia (HHT)

Rare
- Bloom's syndrome
- Telangiectatic haemangioma (reticular infantile haemangioma)
- Cutis marmorata telangiectatica

- Liver disease
- Osler–Weber–Rendu disease
- Ataxia telangiectasia
- Generalised essential telangiectasia
- Topical steroid treatment
- CREST syndrome
- Congenital cutis marmorata telangiectatica (CCMT)
- Hereditary benign telangiectasia
- Idiopathic telangiectasia
- Unilateral nevoid telangiectasia
- Chronic sun exposure

Differential diagnosis at a glance

	Spider angioma	Pregnancy/oestrogen treatment	Liver disease	Connective tissue diseases	HHT
Effect of oestrogen	Yes	Yes	Yes	No	No
Associated with haemorrhage	No	No	Yes	No	Yes
Inherited	No	No	No	Possible	Yes
Visceral involvement	No	No	Yes	Possible	Yes
Benign	Yes	Yes	No	No	No

Recommended investigations

***   Urinalysis to exclude renal disease in collagen diseases (e.g. systemic lupus erythematosus (SLE)).

***   LFT for suspected liver disease.

***   Immunoglobulin to exclude syndromes associated with immunoglobulin deficiency.

**   Pregnancy test may be needed for widespread telangiectasia and in case of spider angiomas.

***   ANA and SLE double-strand test to exclude SLE for connective tissue diseases.

**   X-rays of legs may detect calcinosis in CREST syndrome.

TOP TIPS

◪ Spider angiomas (nevus araneus) are a very common condition, occurring in up to 15% of pre-school-age children and 45% of school-age children. Lesions occur predominately on the face and dorsa of the hands. They often disappear in children and tend to persist in adults.

◪ Telangiectasia is a part of an important syndrome: CREST (calcinosis, Raynaud's syndrome, oesophageal, sclerodactyly and telangiectasia). Two or more of these features establish the diagnosis.

◪ Soon after children begin to walk, ataxia telangiectasia manifests as progressive cerebellar ataxia, sino-pulmonary symptoms, and immunodeficiency. Children are wheelchair bound usually aged 10–12 years. Telangiectasia appears at 3–6 years of age.

◪ Bloom's syndrome, inherited as an autosomal recessive on chromosome 15, manifests usually in infancy as erythema and telangiectasia on the face in a butterfly distribution, similar to SLE, after sun exposure.

◪ By far the most common cause of telangiectasia is the 'normal telangiectasia' appearing on the cheeks of healthy children. They should not be linked to any disease such as liver disease.

◪ Some telangiectasia are not obvious and need to be searched for, e.g. in the bulbar conjunctive in ataxia telangiectasia and on the tongue and mucous membranes in hereditary haemorrhagic telangiectasia.

- Majority of cases with cutis marmorata are trivial and occur commonly in neonates and infants. More pronounced and persistent lesions during exercise, crying and changes of environmental temperature could well be due to CCMT. This is also benign.

- Although spider angiomas commonly occur in healthy children, they may occur in association with pregnancy and liver disease. Therefore, individuals may need to be tested for these conditions.
- Beware that children with HHT often experience recurrent epistaxis, and other haemorrhages (gastrointestinal, mouth and lungs) before the typical telangiectasia, which usually develops at puberty.
- Although Raynaud's phenomenon is often benign, and due to reactive peripheral vasoconstriction, some children do develop later connective tissue disease, particularly progressive systemic sclerosis and CREST syndrome. Screening them with ANAs is useful.
- HHT is one of the many causes of stroke. Around 15%–20% of patients with pulmonary arteriovenous malformation present with stroke due to embolic abscesses.

NOTES:

EXCESSIVE SWEATING (HYPERHIDROSIS)

The clinician overview

Eccrine sweat glands, found all over the skin's surface, cool the body through the evaporation of sweat. Apocrine sweat glands, mainly present in the axillae, anogenital skin and mammary areas, produce viscous fluid to give the body a distinctive odour. Excessive perspiration due to overactive sweat glands can be generalised or localised to certain parts of the body such as palms, axillae or soles of the feet. It can also be primary (usually idiopathic) or secondary, caused by an underlying condition (e.g. hyperthyroidism). Excessive sweating is a common problem and can be distressing, leading to embarrassment and avoidance of social contact.

Possible diagnoses

INFANTS
Common
- Warm environment
- Infection
- Drugs (antipyretics)
- Warmly dressed
- Excessive crying

Rare
- Heart failure

CHILDREN

- Fever (phase of defervescence)
- Emotion/anxiety
- Endocrine (e.g. hyperthyroidism, hypoglycaemia)
- Idiopathic (primary, which is genetic)
- Obesity

- Drugs (e.g. antidepressants, omeprazole, antipyretics)
- Rickets
- Exercise
- Heart failure
- Familial dysautonomia
- Malignancy (e.g. lymphoma)
- TB
- Withdrawal from narcotics, opiates
- Carcinoid syndrome
- Cord transaction
- Chédiak–Higashi syndrome

Differential diagnosis at a glance

	Fever	Emotion/anxiety	Endocrine	Idiopathic	Obesity
Generalised	Yes	No	Yes	Possible	No
Profuse	Yes	Possible	Possible	Possible	Possible
Ill-looking	Possible	No	Possible	No	No
Associated pallor	No	Possible	No	No	No
Diagnosis obvious	Yes	Possible	No	No	Yes

Recommended investigations

The vast majority of cases with hyperhidrosis do not require investigation, as the cause is clinically clear.

***   Blood glucose for suspected cases of hypoglycaemia.
***   TFTs will confirm hyperthyroidism.
***   Serological tests for chronic diseases such as brucellosis.
***   Chest X-ray to search for lymphoma.

TOP TIPS

- In children with acute hyperhidrosis, defervescence after fever is by far the most common cause.
- The low self-esteem and social isolation experienced by some patients with hyperhidrosis may be compounded by the malodorous (bromhidrosis) and fetid odour caused by decomposition of the sweat by bacteria and yeasts.
- Primary hyperhidrosis begins around puberty and tends to be localised in the axillae, hands, face and the soles of the feet. It is a lifelong problem.
- As primary hyperhidrosis is a lifelong problem, clinicians have an important role in supporting affected children by explaining that there is nothing wrong with them and encouraging them to adhere to hygienic measures (bathing and changing clothes daily), using regular antiperspirants and avoiding foods that stimulate sweating such as coffee, spicy food and onions.
- Aluminium hydrochloride as a 20% solution is often helpful in excessive sweating confined to the palms and soles of the feet.

- Beware that in severe cases of sweating, the skin, especially on the feet, may be macerated, fissured and scaling. This can be mistakenly diagnosed as a primary infection such as fungal infection rather than sweating as the primary cause. On the other hand, increased hydration may contribute to pyogenic infection and contact dermatitis.
- In cases of unexplained generalised sweating, diseases such as hyperthyroidism, hypoglycaemia, TB, brucellosis or lymphoma may be the underlying systemic cause.
- Don't forget that episodic sweating, particularly if associated with abdominal symptoms (diarrhoea, vomiting or pain), could have carcinoid syndrome or phaeochromocytoma as an underlying cause.
- Although transthoracic sympathectomy offers the only permanent cure for patients with severe hyperhidrosis, symptom recurrences, pneumothorax and compensatory hyperhidrosis (excessive sweating elsewhere) may occur after this intervention.

NOTES:

Unexplained fever

Fever without focus

Prolonged fever (PUO)

Recurrent fever (periodic and relapsing fever)

Postoperative fever

Recurrent febrile infection

FEVER WITHOUT FOCUS

The clinician overview

Fever without focus (FWF) is defined as an acute febrile illness without apparent source that lasts for less than a week, with the history and physical examination having failed to find the cause. About 20% of all febrile episodes demonstrate no localising signs on presentation. The most common cause is a viral infection, mostly occurring during the first few years of life. Such an infection should be considered only after excluding urinary tract infection and bacteraemia. Bacteraemia indicates the presence of bacteria in the blood, while septicaemia suggests tissue invasion by the bacteria, causing tissue hypoperfusion and organ dysfunction. Neonates and young infants, ill-appearing children and those with impaired immunity more often have septicaemia rather than bacteraemia. Clinicians facing a case of FWF are challenged to decide what laboratory tests are indicated, who can be sent home safely and who should be hospitalised and treated with antibiotics.

Possible diagnoses

INFANTS
Common
- Maternal fever
- Viral infection
- Urinary tract infection (UTI)
- Occult bacteraemia
- Occult abscess

Rare
- Drug fever
- Pneumonia
- Malaria
- Recurrent fevers (other than malaria)
- Meningitis

CHILDREN
- Viral infection (e.g. human herpesvirus-6 (HHV-6))
- UTI
- Occult bacteraemia
- Juvenile rheumatoid arthritis (JRA)
- Malaria

- Drug fever
- Pneumonia
- Sinusitis
- Recurrent fevers (other than malaria)
- Occult abscess
- Dengue fever

Differential diagnosis at a glance

	Viral infection	UTI	Occult bacteraemia	JRA	Malaria
Hectic, high fever with rigour	No	Possible	Possible	Possible	Possible
Fever has a diagnostic pattern	No	No	No	Yes	Yes
Ill-appearing	No	Possible	Yes	Possible	Possible
Often female sex	No	Yes	No	Yes	No
Leukocytosis and high CRP	No	Yes	Yes	Yes	Possible

Recommended investigation

***   Urine: dipsticks may show positive nitrite that is highly sensitive for UTI.

***   FBC: leukocytosis and high CRP suggest bacterial infection such as bacteraemia or UTI.

***   BC: for highly febrile children (> 39°C) aged over 3 months, any ill child or child younger than 3 months.

***   ANA: for JRA, a negative is more important in excluding JRA than a positive in suggesting JRA.

***   Thick and thin peripheral film for suspected malaria.

**   Abdominal ultrasound scan looking for any hidden abscess.

TOP TIPS

- Viral infections are the causes of fever in 90%–95% of cases in general and in 40%–60% in fever without focus. It is the clinician's role to identify a bacterial cause in those children who may need antibiotics.

- Children with a viral infection are likely to appear well, with good eye contact, a reasonable level of activity, not dehydrated and eating and drinking satisfactorily.

- Exanthema subitum (caused by HHV-6) is the most common febrile exanthem in children younger than 3 years, occurring in about 30% of children. Onset of fever is abrupt (sometimes triggering a febrile seizure) and characteristically continuous, often as high as 40°C–41°C and without a focus. The temperature usually drops by crisis coinciding with the appearance of the rash. Characteristically, the child becomes well and afebrile when the rash erupts.

- Children aged 3–24 months have the highest incidence of bacteraemia, estimated to be 3%–4% with children aged 7–12 months having twice the incidence of those aged 13–18 months.

- While the risk of bacteraemia is negligible with temperatures of 38°C–39°C, a strong correlation exists between the incidence of bacteraemia and higher temperatures: it is 7%

with temperatures of 40–40.5°C, 13% with 40.5°C–41.0°C and 26% with a temperature higher than 41.0°C.

☑ Although bacteraemia occurs more often as a primary isolated disease, meningitis is associated with positive blood culture in 50%–80%, pneumonia in about 10% and otitis media 1.5%.

☑ Abnormal findings in children with bacteraemia are usually absent, with ill appearance being the only manifestations of the disease. Occult bacteraemia may be associated with well appearance.

☑ Although viral infections account for the vast majority of causes of fever (90%–95%), children younger than 3 months of age, those with immune deficiency (e.g. HIV or on chemotherapy), sickle-cell anaemia (SCA), cystic fibrosis (CF), asplenia and with body temperature higher than 41°C should be considered as having bacterial infections until proven otherwise, and treatment with antibiotics should be commenced without waiting for the laboratory results.

☑ Infants younger than 3 months of age and ill-appearing infants and children should be hospitalised, their urine and blood cultured (lumbar puncture is often performed as well) and should receive IV ceftriaxone or cefotaxime. Older children with fever higher than 39.0°C should be screened with blood WBC and CRP; if elevated, treatment with ceftriaxone or cefotaxime should be initiated while waiting for the BC result.

☑ A viral infection should be considered only after excluding bacterial infection, such as urinary tract infection (UTI) and bacteraemia. UTI can almost certainly be excluded by urine dipsticks (negative WBC and nitrite). Once UTI has been excluded, bacteraemia should be considered. High fever, leukocytosis and high CRP suggest the bacterial aetiology.

☑ Although occult bacteraemia occurs in about 3%–4% of rather well-appearing febrile children, neonates and small infants often manifest with life-threatening septicaemia.

☑ Always remember that normal body temperature does not preclude serious bacterial infection.

NOTES:

PROLONGED FEVER OF UNKNOWN ORIGIN

The clinician overview

Prolonged fever of unknown origin (PUO) is defined as fever without localising signs that persists for 1 week during which evaluation in the hospital fails to detect the cause. Infections are the most common causes, accounting for 60%–70% of all cases. The younger the child, the higher the relative percentage of infection. Although the majority of viral infections rarely cause prolonged fever, about 15% of the infectious cases of PUO are due to viral infection. Collagen diseases account for about 20%, of which the most common cause is juvenile rheumatoid arthritis (JRA) as a pre-arthritic presentation. Malignancy presenting as fever without other manifestations is unusual in children compared with the rate in adults, but may occur in up to 5%. Miscellaneous diagnoses account for 5%–10% and undiagnosed in the remaining 5%. Previously, a high percentage of PUO (up to 25%) was categorised as undiagnosed, but with recently developed techniques, in particular imaging, the percentage of undiagnosed cases has greatly decreased.

Possible diagnoses

INFANTS
Common
- Bacterial infection (e.g. TB, brucellosis)
- Collagen-vascular (e.g. JRA, systemic lupus erythematosus (SLE))
- Viral (e.g. cytomegalovirus (CMV), Epstein–Barr virus (EBV))
- Hereditary (e.g. Anhidrotic ectodermal dysplasia)
- Parasitic infections

Rare
- Some cases of periodic fever (e.g. familial Mediterranean fever)
- Induced illness by proxy
- Rickettsia

CHILDREN
- Bacterial infection (e.g. brucellosis, mycoplasma)
- Collagen-vascular (e.g. JRA, SLE, Kawasaki's disease)
- Viral (e.g. CMV, EBV, HIV)
- Parasitic infection (e.g. malaria, toxoplasmosis)
- Neoplasms

- Drug fever
- Rickettsia
- Subacute thyroiditis (de Quervain's disease)
- Periodic and relapsing fever
- Lyme disease
- Inflammatory bowel disease
- Factitious fever

Diagnosis at a glance

	Bacterial infection	Collagen-vascular	Viral	Parasitic infection	Neoplasms
Child relatively well	Possible	Possible	Yes	Possible	No
Associated weight loss	Possible	Possible	No	Possible	Yes
Mostly occurring in tropics	Possible	No	No	Yes	No
May respond to an antibiotic trial	Yes	No	No	Possible	No
Leukocytosis, high CRP, ESR	Yes	Possible	No	Possible	Possible

Recommended investigation

The tempo of laboratory investigation is based on the child's condition, while the extent of investigation is based on clues obtained from history.

*** Urine for dipstick testing, microscopy and culture.

*** FBC, CRP, ESR, blood film, BC.

** Stool: microscopy and culture (WBC > 5RBC/hpf suggests bacterial aetiology).

*** Tuberculin test.

** Lumbar puncture (if history or physical examination suspects an infection).

** LFTs, serum albumin: globulin ratio.

** ANA for JRA.

** Viral studies.

** Serology for brucellosis, toxoplasmosis, CMV, EBV, salmonella.

** Chest X-ray for TB? CT scan for sinuses; ultrasound scan of abdomen for any occult abscess.

** Echocardiography for vegetation in endocarditis, if a cardiac murmur is present.

** Isotope bone scan: to look for any osteomyelitic focus or tumour.

TOP TIPS

◪ The patient's history should be searched for animal exposure, travel abroad, prior use of antibiotics, ingestion of raw milk, exposure to infection and consideration of ethnic group.

◪ Repeated physical examinations are more helpful in establishing a diagnosis than extensive investigations.

◪ A child with the initial diagnosis of PUO on presentation may often prove to have either a self-limiting benign disorder, such as viral infection (fever being the only sign of the disease), or a common disease with atypical presentation (such as lymphoma or SLE). PUO caused by JRA occurs during the non-arthritic paucity of symptoms and with fever being the only sign.

- With the exception of bone marrow aspiration, invasive techniques, such as laparotomy, laparoscopy or biopsy are rarely indicated nowadays to diagnose PUO. Rheumatoid arthritis in a child with an established diagnosis of PUO is often the single most common diagnosis.
- The prognosis of PUO is better in children than in adults, mainly because of the higher incidence of infection and lower incidence of malignancy. Fatality may occur in less than 5% of the patients primarily due to neoplastic causes.
- Fever of neoplastic origin usually does not respond to antipyretics such as paracetamol but does respond to indomethacin or naproxen. Naproxen causes a prompt and complete lysis of neoplastic fever with sustained normal temperature (Naproxen test). Naproxen is therefore useful in the differential diagnosis between neoplastic and infectious fevers.

Red flags

- Beware that an absence of sweat with high fever may suggest heat stroke, dehydration, anhidrotic ectodermal dysplasia or familial dysautonomia. The latter is associated with lack of tears, absent corneal reflex and smooth tongue.
- Careful palpating of muscles and bones may suggest occult osteomyelitis or bone marrow invasion by tumour.
- Eye examination by an ophthalmologist is essential and may suggest the diagnosis: bulbar conjunctivitis suggests Kawasaki's disease or leptospirosis; palpebral conjunctivitis may suggest TB, glandular fever or cat-scratch fever; petechial conjunctival haemorrhage suggests endocarditis; uveitis is an early clue for JRA or sarcoidosis; chorioretinitis suggests toxoplasmosis, syphilis or CMV.
- Factitious fever, although rare, is an important cause of PUO (incidence 1%–2% of causes of PUO). Measurement of temperature by a nurse attending to the procedure is essential to eliminate the rare possibility.

NOTES:

RECURRENT FEVER (PERIODIC AND RELAPSING FEVER)

The clinician overview

Periodic fever (PF) and relapsing fever (ReF) are characterised by episodes of fever recurring at regular or irregular intervals; each episode is followed by one to several days, weeks or months of normal temperature. Examples are seen in malaria, brucellosis, familial Mediterranean fever (FMF) and PFAPA (periodic fever, aphthous stomatitis, pharyngitis, and cervical adenitis). RF is recurrent fever caused by numerous species of *Borrelia* and transmitted by lice (louse-borne RF) or ticks (tick-borne RF). Familial cold urticaria syndrome (FCUS), Muckle–Wells syndrome (MWS), TNF-receptor associated periodic syndrome (TRAPS) and hyperimmunoglobulinaemia D syndrome (HIDS) are also characterised by recurrent episodes of fever but they are rare compared with FMF.

Possible diagnoses

INFANTS
Common
- ☑ FMF
- ☑ Brucellosis
- ☑ Malaria
- ☑ MWS
- ☑ Cyclic neutropenia

Rare
- ☑ FCUS
- ☑ TRAPS
- ☑ MWS
- ☑ HIDS

CHILDREN
- ☑ Malaria
- ☑ Brucellosis
- ☑ FMF
- ☑ PFAPA
- ☑ Cyclic neutropenia

- ☑ FCUS

Diagnosis at a glance

	Malaria	FMF	Brucellosis	PFAPA	Cyclic neutropenia
Inheritance either autosomal dominant or recessive	No	Yes	No	Yes	Yes
Periodicity of fever 3–6 weeks	No	Yes	No	Yes	Yes
Mouth ulcers	No	No	No	Yes	Yes
Myalgia/arthralgia	Yes	Yes	Yes	No	No
Prevalent in Mediterranean area	Possible	Yes	Yes	No	No

Recommended investigation

***   FBC: neutropenia < 1000 will confirm cyclic neutropenia.

***   IgD is elevated in HIDS and in the majority of cases of PFAPA.

***   Giemsa-stained smear for malaria, serological test for brucellosis.

**   CRP and ESR: usually elevated.

TOP TIPS

◪ Genetic causes of periodic fever syndromes have been identified in the past few years. The term autoinflammatory disease has been proposed to describe a group of disorders characterised by attacks of unprovoked systemic inflammation without significant levels of autoimmune or infective causes.

◪ FMF occurs in individuals from Mediterranean ancestry who usually present with loss of appetite and abdominal pain due to peritonitis. About 6–10 hours later, fever occurs and rapid recovery ensues within 24–72 hours.

◪ Episodes of PFAPA are the most common clinical features of autoinflammatory disease. Each episode is followed by a symptom-free interval ranging from weeks to months.

◪ Patients with FMF usually respond dramatically to colchicine at 0.6 mg hourly for 4 doses, which is also effective in preventing attacks of FMF and the development of amyloidosis. For those with PFAPA, steroid therapy is very effective in controlling fever and other symptoms within 2–4 hours. IgD is elevated in the majority of cases of PFAPA.

◪ Amyloidosis commonly complicates FMF. Proteinuria is often the clue to the disease. The best site to confirm the diagnosis is a biopsy from the gingiva or rectum, not from the kidney or spleen.

◪ Cyclic neutropenia, autosomal dominant, is characterised by pharyngitis, mouth ulcers, lymphadenitis and fever regularly occurring at 3-week intervals. Beware that neutropenia may be associated with septicaemia.

Red flags

- Pel–Ebstein fever was originally thought to be characteristic of Hodgkin's lymphoma (HL). Only a few patients with Hodgkin's disease develop this pattern, but when present, this is an important clue for the presence of HL. The pattern consists of recurrent episodes of fever lasting 3–10 days, followed by an afebrile period of similar duration.
- The resolution of a febrile episode in periodic fever may be accompanied within a few hours (6–8 hours) by the Jarisch–Herxheimer reaction (JHR), which usually follows antibiotic treatment. The reaction is caused by the release of endotoxin when the organisms are destroyed by antibiotics. JHR is very common after treating patients with syphilis.

NOTES:

POSTOPERATIVE FEVER

The clinician overview

Postoperative fever is defined as a temperature greater than 38°C on two consecutive postoperative days, or 39°C on any postoperative day. Fever during the postoperative period is common, occurring in 25%–50% of cases. The magnitude of fever is correlated with the extent of the surgery, i.e. minor surgery is rarely associated with fever. Early postoperative fever (within 48 hours postoperatively) is often caused by the trauma of the surgery. Infection is the cause of fever in about 10%–25% of febrile postoperative patients, usually occurring after 48 hours, lasting longer than 2 days (unless treated with antibiotics) and higher than 39°C, and is associated with ill appearance.

Possible diagnoses

INFANTS
Common
- Dehydration
- High ambient temperature
- Septicaemia
- Intravenous line infection
- Haematoma

Rare
- Infectious diarrhoea
- Urinary tract infection (UTI)
- Osteomyelitis
- Pulmonary atelectasis

CHILDREN

- Dehydration
- Wound infection
- Transfusion or drug reaction
- Haematoma
- Pneumonia

- UTI
- Bacteraemia

Diagnosis at a glance

	Dehydration	Wound infection	Transfusion or drug reaction	Haematoma	Pneumonia
High fever (> 39.0°C)	No	Possible	Possible	No	Yes
Fever appears on day 1 of surgery	Yes	No	Possible	Possible	No
Ill appearance	Possible	Possible	Possible	Possible	Yes
Diagnosis by seeing the surgery site	No	Yes	No	Yes	No
Leukocytosis with high CRP	No	Yes	Possible	No	Yes

Recommended investigation

***   Urine dipstick testing and culture in every case.

***   FBC and CRP: high levels suggest bacterial infection.

***   LFT; if clinically indicated, e.g. in the presence of jaundice, abdominal pain.

***   BC if fever is > 39.0°C, and/or FBC and CRP are high.

***   Chest X-ray, in particular if pneumonia is clinically suspected.

**   Viral studies: occasionally requested if the fever persists.

***   CT scan and/or ultrasonography: sometimes required for detecting intra-abdominal abscess.

TOP TIPS

- Physical examination should focus on sites most likely to be the cause of fever, including the operative site, abdomen (for distension, tenderness, absence of bowel sounds) and upper respiratory tract for infection and lung auscultation.
- The diagnosis of non-infectious causes should only be considered after excluding infectious causes.
- Factors that increase the likelihood of infection include a long postoperative stay in hospital, fever commencing on the third postoperative day or later and fever over 39°C that persists or has a hectic pattern, and the presence of an intravascular catheter, the prolonged use of a naso-gastric or endotracheal tube, indwelling urinary catheter or shunt.
- Before embarking on performing tests for postoperative fever, remember that the most common source of infectious fever is wound infection.

- Beware that serious infection may exist in the absence of fever; this is usually the case during the neonatal period and in immunosuppressed children.
- The importance of postoperative fever is because of the possibility of infection, which can lead to death if not properly treated.
- Although most postoperative fevers are non-infectious, patients should be treated with antibiotics if they appear unwell, the source of the fever is obscured or there is leukocytosis with high CRP. These suggest infections which may be serious and life-threatening.

NOTES:

RECURRENT FEBRILE INFECTION

The clinician overview

Recurrent infections are a source of great concern to parents and primary care clinicians, and a common reason to bring children for medical advice. The term refers to infections that are too frequent, severe or long-lasting. It has been estimated that normal young children may have as many as 12–16 recurrent infections per year if they attend nursery, nine infections per year if a sibling attends school, and six or eight per year if the child and a sibling are not at school. Respiratory tract and diarrhoeal infections are the most common diseases. Fortunately, the rate of these infections decline as the child grows older.

Possible diagnoses

INFANTS

Common
- Prematurity
- Infants younger than 3 months
- Maternal infections
- Hospitalisation
- Central venous line

Rare
- Malnutrition
- Neutropenia and lymphopenia
- Immunodeficiency
- Asplenia
- Wiskott-Aldrich syndrome
- Malignancy
- SCA

CHILDREN

- Normal (particularly those attending daycare centres)
- Immunodeficiency
- Sickle-cell anaemia (SCA)
- Neutropenia and lymphopenia
- Malnutrition

- Asplenia
- Drugs (e.g. oral steroids)
- DiGeorge syndrome (thymic hypoplasia)
- Malignancy
- Wiskott–Aldrich syndrome
- Ataxia telangiectasia

Diagnosis at a glance

	Normal	Immunodeficiency	SCA	Neutropenia and lymphopenia	Malnutrition
Infections usually viral	Yes	No	No	No	No
Associated underweight	No	Possible	Possible	Possible	Possible
+ family history	No	Possible	Possible	Possible	Possible
Improve when getting older	Yes	No	No	Possible	Possible
Abnormal FBC (Hb, WBC)	No	Yes	Yes	Yes	Possible

Recommended investigation

***   Urine: for culture.

***   FBC: looking for neutrophil and lymphocyte counts.

***   Immunoglobulins.

**   Chest: X-ray or ultrasound scan to assess the presence and size of the thymus.

TOP TIPS

◪ Children with mainly or only viral infections (seen in children attending daycare centres) are unlikely to have an immunodeficiency.

◪ As children in daycare centres receive frequent and prolonged courses of antibiotics, resistance to antibiotics has become an alarming problem.

◪ Nosocomial infections (those acquired during hospitalisation) affect 3%–5% of children admitted to hospital. The rate is higher in intensive care units and emergency and long-term care departments.

◪ Primary immunodeficiency diseases (B- and T-cell diseases) are rare except the selective IgA deficiency (all other immunoglobulins are normal), which has a frequency of 1 per 333.

◪ Normal absolute neutrophil and lymphocyte counts alone eliminate most causes of immunodeficiency.

◪ The majority of children (90%–95%) who present with recurrent infections do not have identifiable immunodeficiency; the cause is likely to be frequent exposure to microorganisms in daycare centres or school.

- Beware drug-induced neutropenia remains one of the most common causes of neutropenia; it increases with age from 10% in children to 50% in adults. Neutropenia can cause serious infection.
- Remember that cyclic neutropenia occurs periodically every 3 weeks. During the neutropenia, patients often suffer from stomatitis, oral ulcers, fever and lymphadenopathy. Without symptoms, neutrophil count may be normal.

NOTES:

Urinary

Blood in urine (haematuria)

Painful urination (dysuria)

Frequent urination

Excessive urination (polyuria)

Incontinence of urine (daytime or diurnal)

Bedwetting (nocturnal enuresis)

Urine retention and failure to pass urine

BLOOD IN URINE (HAEMATURIA)

The clinician overview

Gross haematuria indicates that blood is seen with the naked eye. Microhaematuria is more common (incidence 1%–2% of school-age children) and is defined as > 5RBC/hpf in the urine sediment of centrifuged freshly voided urine. In contrast to gross haematuria, the majority of patients (about 80%) with microhaematuria have no clinically identifiable cause for the haematuria. The haematuria of glomerular disease is usually uniformly red with proteinuria and casts but without clots or pain. An exception is Henöch–Schönlein purpura (HSP), which is associated with significant abdominal pain. Haematuria associated with pain may also suggest urolithiasis, urinary tract infection (UTI) or renal tumour. When parents seek medical attention because of blood in urine, doctors should be aware that not all red urine is necessarily blood. Red urine may be due to drugs (e.g. rifampicin, nitrofurantoin), organic biochemicals (e.g. porphyrins, methaemoglobin), pigments (e.g. haemoglobin, myoglobin) or food (e.g. beets, blackberries).

Possible diagnoses

INFANTS
Common

- Asphyxia
- Renal vein thrombosis (cross haematuria)
- Blood dyscrasias
- Drugs
- Infection (sepsis)
- Obstructive uropathy

Rare

- Coagulopathy (e.g. thrombocytopenia)
- Tumour (e.g. nephroblastoma)
- Trauma
- Renal artery thrombosis
- Cortical and medullary necrosis

CHILDREN

- IgA nephropathy
- Poststreptococcal glomerulonephritis (PSGN)
- UTI: bacteria, parasitic (e.g. schistosomiasis), viral (e.g. adenovirus), bacterial (e.g. *E. coli*)
- HSP
- Bladder/urethral bleeding

- Coagulopathy (e.g. thrombocytopenia, haemophilia)
- Systemic lupus erythematosus (SLE)
- Vascular (e.g. renal vein thrombosis, sickle-cell anaemia)
- Haemolytic-uraemic syndrome (HUS)
- Renal stones

- ☑ Idiopathic haematuria
- ☑ Tumour (e.g. nephroblastoma, bladder hamartoma)
- ☑ Alport's syndrome
- ☑ Polycystic kidneys
- ☑ Goodpasture syndrome (associated with pulmonary haemorrhage)
- ☑ Drugs (e.g. cyclophosphamide)
- ☑ Hypercalciuria
- ☑ Haemorrhagic cystitis (cyclophosphamide)
- ☑ High-intensity exercise
- ☑ Wegener's granulomatosis
- ☑ Nutcracker syndrome (compressed left renal vein)

Differential diagnosis at a glance

	IgA nephropathy	PSGN	UTI	HSP	Bladder/ urethral bleeding
Abdominal pain	No	No	Possible	Yes	Possible
Protein, casts	Yes	Yes	Possible	Yes	No
High serum C3	No	Yes	No	No	No
History of URTI/ tonsillitis	Possible	Yes	No	Possible	No
High blood pressure and, creatinine	No	Yes	No	Possible	No
Recurrent	Yes	No	Possible	Possible	Possible

Recommended investigations

***   Urine dipstick testing confirms the RBCs; proteinuria suggests that haematuria is renal in origin; the presence of RBC casts indicates glomerulonephritis.

***   24-hour urine collection for calcium excretion (abnormal if > 4 mg/kg), or for the extent of proteinuria.

***   FBC: anaemia in HUS, haemolytic anaemia, chronic renal disease; leucopenia in SLE, thrombocytopenia in SLE; reticulocytosis in haemolytic anaemia.

***   High antistreptolysin titre (or better streptozyme if available) suggests PSGN.

***   U&E: increased creatinine and urea in HUS and chronic renal failure. Calcium to rule out hypercalcaemia.

*** Complement levels: low but recover in 6–8 weeks in PSGN, and persistent in proliferative glomerulonephritis (GN).

*** Autoantibodies (ANF, anti-double-stranded DNA antibody for immune-mediated GN).

*** Renal ultrasound scan: provide in hydronephrosis, calculus, tumour and calcification.

*** Cystoscopy for bladder source of bleeding, e.g. haemangiomas, or from lesion in the ureter.

*** In tropics search for schistosomiasis haematobium eggs in urine and faeces.

TOP TIPS

◪ Haematuria on dipstick testing always needs confirmation by microscopy.

◪ Microscopic haematuria is common and transient in healthy children. Persistent microscopic haematuria indicates the presence of > 5RBC/hpf microscopically detected at monthly intervals.

◪ Isolated microscopic haematuria is either idiopathic or due to hypercalciuria (in 25% of cases). In the latter, hypercalcaemic hypercalciuria needs to be excluded by checking serum calcium.

◪ Gross haematuria may be either associated with mild oedema, hypertension, oliguria and renal failure (nephritic syndrome), or gross oedema and proteinuria (nephrotic syndrome).

◪ In contrast to microscopic haematuria, evaluation of gross haematuria usually yields positive findings that will establish the diagnosis.

◪ IgA nephropathy is the most common cause of recurrent painless haematuria; typical age is 8–10 years. Gross haematuria subsides soon to be followed by microscopic haematuria.

◪ The most common cause of gross haematuria worldwide is PSGN. The urine is uniformly red, brownish-red or dark brown (Coca-Cola colour), which usually contains RBCs casts.

◪ Remember that proteinuria in association with haematuria is very suggestive of the renal origin of blood. The presence of casts, particularly RBCs casts, indicates glomerulonephritis.

◪ Beware that although UTI is usually caused by bacterial infection, common respiratory virus, adenovirus, can cause haemorrhagic cystitis, particularly in immunocompromised status.

◪ Normal serum levels of C3 in IgA nephropathy distinguishes this disorder from PSGN.

◪ One of the most common causes of gross haematuria is hypercalciuria without renal stones. This can be confirmed by elevated calcium excretion of > 4 mg/kg in 24-hour urine collection.

◪ Urolithiasis may develop from hypercalciuria; the risk is higher in cases of gross haematuria.

◪ Recurrent episodes of gross haematuria following an upper respiratory tract infection are a common presentation of IgA nephropathy. Diagnosis is established not by serum complement or IgA levels but by renal biopsy showing glomerular IgA immune deposits.

◪ For any degree of haematuria, the imaging of choice is ultrasonography, not a plain X-ray. Malformation, tumours, urolithiasis, nephrocalcinosis can be demonstrated accurately.

◪ In many countries, e.g. Egypt, haematuria is mostly due to *Schistosoma haematobium*. Diagnosis is made by detection of eggs in the urine and faeces, or biopsy of the bladder, rectum or liver.

- Beware that renal tumours may bleed, typically in association with abdominal pain or a palpable mass. An urgent ultrasound scan should be performed.
- Do not suggest a diagnosis of UTI based on urine RBCs or protein or both. Positive nitrite and WBCs in the dipstick are more specific and sensitive for UTI than blood and protein.
- While adults and older children with urolithiasis nearly always present with severe flank pain and haematuria, pre-school children usually present with UTI, a less-severe degree of flank pain and haematuria. An urgent ultrasound scan is needed to establish the diagnosis.

NOTES:

PAINFUL URINATION (DYSURIA)

The clinician overview

Dysuria is often accompanied by other urinary symptoms such as frequency, urgency or hesitancy. Although this can sometimes be a sign of urinary tract infection (UTI), it is more commonly caused by vulvovaginitis, balanitis or urethritis. The majority of cases of dysuria are self-limiting and identified by physical examination with urine or discharge cultures. Children sometimes express itching as dysuria, and this is commonly seen with worm infestation. Persistent dysuria with a normal examination and negative urine cultures are likely to be due to dysfunctional void or hypercalciuria.

Possible diagnoses

INFANTS
Common
- Nappy rash (diaper dermatitis)
- Meatal ulceration
- Atopic dermatitis
- Balanitis
- Chemical irritation

Rare
- Herpes simplex infection (peri-urethral)
- Varicella (peri-urethral lesions)

CHILDREN
- UTI (mainly lower UTI)
- Vulvovaginitis
- Balanitis
- STD
- Urethritis/cystitis

- Reiter's syndrome
- Sexual abuse
- Drugs
- Hypercalciuria (dysuria with haematuria)
- Herpes simplex infection
- Labial adhesions
- Pinworms
- Lichen planus
- Stevens–Johnson syndrome

Differential diagnosis at a glance

	UTI	Vulvovaginitis	Balanitis	STD	Urethritis/cystitis
Most common	Yes	Yes	No	No	No
+ urine culture	Yes	Possible	No	Possible	Possible
Fever	Yes	No	No	No	Possible
Bacterial infection	Yes	Possible	Possible	Yes	Possible
Discharge	No	Possible	Possible	Yes	Possible

Recommended investigations

***	Urinalysis is essential for all cases with dysuria.
***	Children with UTI should be investigated according to the NICE (National Institute for Health and Clinical Excellence) guidelines.
***	Culture of any discharge in girls with vulvovaginitis to exclude infection, or STD.
***	Larvae or ova of threadworms from discharge of vulvovaginitis.
***	Renal ultrasound scan for cases with UTI.

TOP TIPS

◪ In children with dysuria, history and examination will determine whether any test is necessary.

◪ Nappy rash (diaper dermatitis) is the most common cause of dysuria in infancy. This is expressed as crying or discomfort during urination.

◪ Urine dipstick testing is very helpful in suggesting or excluding UTI: the presence of positive nitrite with WBC suggests UTI; when both are negative, UTI is very unlikely.

◪ In patients with normal examination and negative cultures, dysuria may well be caused by hypercalciuria. A 24-hour urine collection for calcium is indicated.

Red flags

◪ Painful urination is occasionally a serious problem for it may cause urine retention with subsequent dilation of the urinary tract system.

◪ A child with vulvovaginitis should undergo a careful history to exclude sexual abuse.

◪ Remember that a foreign body, such as a piece of toilet paper, can be trapped in the vagina, causing discharge and dysuria. Careful area inspection is essential.

◪ Beware that pruritis can be expressed as dysuria; threadworms, which normally infest the perianal area, can occasionally spread to the vagina.

- In a female patient with dysuria and abdominal pain, pelvic inflammatory disease (PID) must be ruled out.
- Asymptomatic infections with either Neisseria gonorrhoeae or chlamydia trachomatis may lead to development of PID, which has serious consequences if left untreated.
- A urethral or vaginal discharge in an adolescent is likely caused by an infection with either Neisseria gonorrhoeae or chlamydia trachomatis.
- When herpes simplex causes urethritis, vesicles may be tiny and inapparent; a thorough examination can clinch the diagnosis.
- Beware that in older children, self-exploratory sexual play and masturbation can cause balanitis or vulvovaginitis, even if the history is negative.

NOTES:

FREQUENT URINATION

The clinician overview

The term indicates frequent (more than seven a day in school-age children) voids of small amounts of urine, often associated with urgency. Female children are more affected than males. In infancy, voiding is physiologically frequent, as often as 15–20 times a day, occurring by reflex bladder contraction mediated by sympathetic nerve system (T10–L2) and parasympathetic nerve system (S2–S4). Over time, bladder control is achieved through gradual bladder enlargement, leading to an increase of bladder capacity, cortical inhibition of the reflex bladder contraction and the ability to consciously tighten the external sphincter to prevent incontinence. In paediatrics, the most common cause is an overactive bladder with or without urinary tract infection (UTI). The condition has to be differentiated from polyuria (in which, although frequent, the amount passed is usually large) and incontinence (which is the involuntary loss of urine).

Possible diagnoses

INFANTS
Common
- Physiological
- Nappy rash (diaper dermatitis)
- Fever

Rare
- Drugs (diuretics)

CHILDREN
- Lower UTI
- Vulvovaginitis
- Overactive bladder (detrusor instability)
- Pollakiuria and anxiety
- Developmental delay (including neurogenic bladder)

- Drugs (diuretics)
- Urethritis (e.g. Reiter's syndrome)
- Ectopic ureter and fistula
- Vaginal voiding
- Bladder outlet obstruction
- Urethral stricture
- Pregnancy
- Excessive intake of caffeine
- Congenital bladder diverticulum

Differential diagnosis at a glance

	Lower UTI	Vulvovaginitis	Overactive bladder	Pollakiuria and anxiety	Developmental delay
With dysuria	Yes	Yes	Yes	Possible	Possible
+ nitrite and WBC	Yes	No	Possible	No	No
Reduced FBC	No	No	Yes	Yes	Yes
More in girls	Yes	Yes	Yes	Possible	No
Fever	Possible	No	No	No	No

Recommended investigation

*** Urinalysis with urine culture.
*** Renal ultrasound scan with pre- and postvoid residual urine estimate.
*** Urodynamic study for neurogenic bladder.

TOP TIPS

- Pollakiuria (from the Greek word 'pollakis' meaning many times) or daytime frequency syndrome of childhood, often occurs as a result of stress-related problems, e.g. anxiety. It is not associated with dysuria or systemic disease. Typical age of occurrence is 4–6 years.
- Dysfunction voiding is a common cause of frequent urination. It is characterised by a void at a smaller than normal amount of urine or a bladder that contracts against a closed sphincter.
- Although vaginal voiding may occur because of ectopic ureter into the vagina, labial adhesions are the most common cause. This occurs typically following urination when the girl experiences incontinence after standing up.
- The most important aspect of frequent urination is to exclude polyuria. Arrange a urine collection over 12 or 24 hours to establish the diagnosis if necessary.
- Ectopic ureter usually occurs in girls and is associated with a duplicate collecting system. This can easily be diagnosed by an ultrasound scan.
- When physical examination and urinalysis are normal, hypercalciuria with or without urolithiasis is often the cause. A 24-hour urine collection for calcium is diagnostic.

Red flags

- Ensure that the frequent voiding is not continuous incontinence; if so, this suggests in boys posterior urethral valve obstruction, and in girls ectopic ureter.

NOTES:

EXCESSIVE URINATION (POLYURIA)

The clinician overview

Excessive loss of body water leads to a rise of plasma osmotic pressure (osmolality), causing thirst and antidiuretic hormone (ADH) release. ADH binds to a receptor, V_2, on the distal tubules and collecting system to increase water reabsorption through cyclic AMP-mediated pathway. This causes increased urine osmolality. Diabetes insipidus (DI) arises if there is no production or release of ADH (e.g. pituitary tumour) or the kidney is unresponsive to the ADH due to mutated V_2 receptor. Other causes of polyuria include osmotic diuresis (diabetes mellitus (DM)), failure of renal tubular concentration ability (Fanconi's syndrome, sickle-cell anaemia (SCA)) or excessive drinking (compulsive drinking). Polyuria is defined as urine output of more than 2 L/m^2 per 24 hours. In general, it results from either a water or solute diuresis. Polyuria must be differentiated from more common complaints of frequency of a small volume of urine. Accurate measurement of 24-hour intake of fluids and quantity of urine excretion should be performed to establish diagnosis of polyuria. Children with polyuria may present with polydipsia, failure to thrive, dehydration, elevated body temperature (hyperthermia), seizure due to hypernatraemic dehydration, and nocturnal enuresis.

Possible diagnoses

INFANTS
Common
- Post-asphyxia

CHILDREN
- DM
- Psychogenic polydipsia (compulsive fluid drinking)
- Renal tubular acidosis (RTA)
- Cranial DI
- Metabolic polyuria (potassium deficiency, hypercalcaemia)

Rare
- Congenital nephrogenic DI

- Congenital and acquired nephrogenic DI
- Sickle-cell anaemia
- Hypercalcaemia
- Chronic renal failure

- ☑ Drugs (diuretics, lithium, chlortetracycline)
- ☑ Drugs affecting renal tubule
- ☑ Renal tubular acidosis (e.g. Fanconi's syndrome)
- ☑ Pituitary tumours (craniopharyngioma, histiocytosis X)
- ☑ Bartter's syndrome
- ☑ Osmotic diuresis

Differential diagnosis at a glance

	DM	Psychogenic polydipsia	Renal tubular acidosis	Cranial DI	Metabolic polyuria
Associated failure to thrive	Possible	No	Yes	Possible	Possible
Short history	Yes	No	No	Possible	Possible
Glycosuria	Yes	No	Yes	No	No
Acidosis	Yes	No	Yes	No	Possible
Hyperglycaemia	Yes	No	No	No	No

Recommended investigations

***   Urinalysis will confirm glycosuria and ketones in DM. Specific gravity: low in DI.

***   Blood glucose (BG), to confirm DM; acid balance and ketones to confirm diabetic ketoacidosis.

***   Osmolality of serum and urine; urine specific gravity.

**   FBC: anaemia is usually present in CRF and SCA.

***   U&E, high creatinine in CRF; low potassium as a cause of polyuria in RTA.

***   Serum calcium: high in hypercalcaemia.

**   ADH serum level estimation in DI: low in cranial DI and normal in nephrogenic DI.

***   MRI for the central causes of DI such as craniopharyngioma.

***   Water deprivation test to differentiate between central and nephrogenic DI.

TOP TIPS

- Although the history and physical examination may provide clues to the causes of polyuria, the definite diagnosis rests on the results of BG, osmolality of the urine and serum, and U&E.
- An isoosmolar (280–300 mOsm/kg) or hyperosmolar (> 300 mOsm/kg) is found in normal children and in solute diuresis, whereas a hypoosmolar urine suggests water diuresis.
- Compulsive thirst can be difficult to differentiate from DI. Hypoosmolar urine and serum suggest compulsive polydipsia; high serum osmolality suggests ADH deficiency or insensitivity.
- It is essential to determine whether the child has frequent, small volume urination or polyuria. Mothers are usually good historians. Observation of the child's urination helps to establish diagnosis.
- Children with compulsive drinking are easily diagnosed by the long history, absence of weight loss or failure to thrive. Low serum osmolality (< 280 mOsm/kg) and urine specific gravity (< 1005) establishes the diagnosis. A specific gravity greater than 1.005 excludes the diagnosis of DI.
- Newly diagnosed diabetics must always be managed at a unit with a specialist paediatrician and nurse.

- Do not miss that the fourth-most-important cause of polyuria is renal tubular acidosis. Children may present with dehydration, failure to thrive, anorexia and vomiting. Diagnosis is easy by finding abnormal biochemical features including glycosuria, low serum bicarbonate and potassium, and hyperchloraemia.
- Beware that nephrogenic DI may present in the first few weeks of life with irritability, poor feeding, failure to gain weight, elevated body temperature and dehydration.
- Although nephrogenic DI occurs virtually only in boys, the female carrier may present with polyuria due to impaired urine concentration ability.
- Urgent investigations and treatment are required for the majority of children with polyuria, particularly DM and DI.
- Unrecognised chronic dehydration, such as that resulting from DI, would lead to hypernatraemia and brain damage.
- Long-standing polyuria may cause enlarged bladder, mega-ureter and hydronephrosis.

NOTES:

INCONTINENCE OF URINE (DAYTIME OR DIURNAL)

The clinician overview

Urinary incontinence is a common problem presenting at primary care services, often associated with nocturnal enuresis (NE). It indicates involuntary loss of urine during the daytime (diurnal) after the age of 5 years. It can be primary (child has been persistently incontinent) or secondary (if the child had achieved a complete dryness for a period of more than 6 months). Primary incontinence rarely has an organic cause and is usually due to developmental delay and genetic causes. Secondary incontinence is usually associated with a stressful event, constipation, diabetes mellitus and child abuse. Incontinence is also classified as neurogenic (congenital or acquired abnormalities of the spinal cord) or, more commonly, non-neurogenic, which is caused by bladder overactivity and anatomical abnormalities.

Possible diagnoses

INFANTS
Common
- Physiological (before 5 years)
- Bladder outlet obstruction
- Lower urinary tract infection (UTI)
- Neurogenic bladder
- Labial adhesions

Rare
- Meningomyelocele
- Ectopic ureter (in girls)
- Sacral anomalies
- Non-neurogenic neurogenic bladder
- Lipomeningocele
- Diabetes insipidus (DI)

CHILDREN
- Unstable bladder (overactive bladder)
- Lower UTI
- Neurogenic bladder
- Giggle incontinence
- Labial adhesions

- Overflow incontinence
- Bladder outlet obstruction (e.g. posterior urethral obstruction)
- Ectopic ureter (in girls)
- Sacral anomalies
- Non-neurogenic neurogenic bladder (detrusor-sphincter dyssynergia = Hinman's syndrome)
- Lipomeningocele
- DI

Differential diagnosis at a glance

	Unstable bladder	Lower UTI	Neurogenic bladder	Giggle incontinence	Labial adhesions
Episodic	No	No	Possible	Yes	No
Frequent urination	Yes	Yes	Possible	No	Yes
Mainly in girls	No	Possible	No	Yes	Yes
+ nitrite and WBC	Possible	Yes	Possible	No	Possible
Examination confirms diagnosis	No	No	Yes	No	Yes

Recommended investigations

***   Urinalysis: positive nitrate and leukocytes suggest UTI, culture will confirm the infection. Specific gravity of urine > 1.005 excludes DI; a 24-hour urine collection is needed to exclude hypercalciuria.

***   Renal ultrasound scan, with pre- and postvoid residual urine estimates, to exclude retention.

***   Urodynamic evaluation may be requested in some cases with neurogenic bladder.

***   Lumbosacral MRI scan is required to diagnose some cases of neurogenic bladder.

TOP TIPS

☑ When parents bring their child for NE, daytime symptoms are usually considered less relevant. Ensure to ask parents and the child about daytime accidents.

☑ Unlike NE, daytime incontinence may often be associated with underlying physical disorders.

☑ While an ectopic ureter usually terminates within the distal third of the vaginal introitus, in boys it usually terminates within the bladder neck or posterior urethra. Therefore, boys do not suffer from incontinence caused by ectopic ureter.

☑ In boys the continuous incontinence is likely to be caused by posterior urethral valves.

☑ Successful management of incontinence includes eliminating caffeine and orange juice from the diet, improving bladder capacity by drinking extra cups of water during the daytime, treating constipation and instructing the child to void regularly every 2–3 hours.

☑ Remember to ask the radiologist on the request form for renal ultrasound to measure the bladder wall thickness: if greater than 5 mm, it indicates a bladder outlet obstruction such as bladder-sphincter dyssynergia in girls and posterior valve in boys.

☑ Daytime incontinence is frequently associated with constipation, faecal soiling and dysfunctional voiding. A careful history will elicit these features.

☑ Daytime incontinence is frequently caused or complicated by UTI. Ensure that a urine sample is examined for UTI each time the child attends the clinic.

- When a girl presents with a history of never gaining urinary control, and underwear is always wet, she probably has ectopic bladder. Confirm the diagnosis by drying the vaginal introitus and inspecting the area every 15 minutes. Re-accumulation of urine is diagnostic.
- Treatment of a child with nighttime and daytime wetting should focus on the daytime problem first. When daytime wetting responds to the treatment, nighttime wetting will improve, not vice versa.

Red flags

- A girl who voids normally but is incontinent day and night has an ectopic ureter until proven otherwise.
- Evaluation of an incontinent child is never complete without inspection of the spine for midline lesions such as hairy patch, buttocks asymmetry or deep sacral dimple. These lesions may be associated with spinal defects such as tethered spinal cord or lipomeningocele.

NOTES:

BEDWETTING (NOCTURNAL ENURESIS)

The clinician overview

Nocturnal enuresis (NE) may present in isolation (monosymptomatic) or associated with daytime wetting, urge symptoms or dysfunctional voiding (complex NE). NE is defined as the involuntary voiding of urine during sleep occurring at least three times a week in a child 5 years of age or older. It is the most common chronic urological disease, affecting over half a million children in the United Kingdom. The incidence at the age of 5 years is about 10%, at the age of 10 years it is around 5% and at puberty 1%–2%. About 15% of children experience a cure annually. Traditionally, NE is divided as primary nocturnal enuresis (PNE), affecting 80% of children, and secondary nocturnal enuresis (SNE), affecting 20% of children. Causes of PNE include genetic (on chromosomes 12 and 13), delayed maturation, sleep disorders and antidiuretic hormone (ADH) deficiency. Causes of SNE include psychogenic, diabetes mellitus (DM), child abuse and diabetes insipidus (DI).

Possible diagnoses

INFANTS
Common

CHILDREN

- PNE
- SNE
- Compulsive fluid drinking
- DM
- Developmental delay

Rare

- Renal tubular acidosis (RTA)
- Renal tubular necrosis
- DI
- Bladder neck obstruction
- Congestive cardiac failure (CCF)
- Chronic renal failure (CRF)

Differential diagnosis at a glance

	PNE	SNE	Compulsive fluid drinking	DM	Developmental delay
+ family history	Possible	Possible	No	Possible	No
Likely psychogenic	No	Yes	Possible	No	No
Associated polydipsia	No	No	Yes	Yes	Possible
Polyuria	No	No	Yes	Yes	No
Short enuresis history	No	Possible	No	Yes	No

Recommended investigations

***   Urine dipstick testing: to screen for infection and glycosuria (DM). Morning urine showing low specific gravity may suggest DI; urine culture to exclude urinary tract infection (UTI).

***   Blood glucose, acid-base analysis, U&E if history suggests DM.

***   Renal ultrasound scan, for children with complex NE, with prevoid and postvoid urine residual estimates. Normal postvoid should not exceed 10% of the prevoid.

TOP TIPS

- A clear urine correlates well with absence of bacteria on dipsticks and with negative urine culture.
- Urinalysis with dipsticks is the most useful screening test to diagnose UTI, DM, RTA (glycosuria without hyperglycaemia). Low specific gravity may suggest DI.
- Children with monosymptomatic NE are unlikely to have an organic disease, and UTI is around 1%. In contrast, those with additional diurnal incontinence have high incidence of UTI and other anatomical abnormalities. Urinalysis is essential at the child's initial visit with both presentations.
- Children with NE have an excellent prognosis: 15% are cured every year.
- Maximal functional bladder capacity (MFBC) is defined by the formula: age of the child × 30 + 30.
- One of the major problems in children with enuresis is low bladder capacity. Ask the parents to measure the amount of the first void in the morning, provided no wetting has occurred at night.
- Nocturia, defined as an amount of urine passed at night which exceeds the MFBC, can be measured by weighing the bed sheet at night. Alternatively, signs such as excessive urine passed (soaking wet), early wetting (in the first 2 hours of sleep), multiple wetting at night and low specific gravity all suggest nocturia.

- Reassuring the child (and parents) that there is overwhelming evidence that he or she will be dry in future, and removing any punishment methods at home are important steps of management.
- A child with PNE will usually need only urine for evaluation; imaging is unnecessary.
- Treatment with desmopressin should mainly be offered for children with evidence of nocturia.

Red flags

- Children presenting with SNE may have a serious underlying disorder such as DM or UTI. Careful history, urinalysis and blood glucose have to be considered.
- Although children at the age of 4 or 5 years with NE may need to be evaluated, active treatment for those under 6 or 7 years is best avoided.
- Beware that one of the presentations of dysfunctional void is non-neurogenic neurogenic bladder (Hinman's syndrome or detrusor-sphincter dyssernergia), which is characterised by failure of the external sphincter to relax during voiding. Children may end with trabeculated bladder, hydronephrosis and renal failure.
- Remember that although lifting a child with NE by the parents is a common practice, this is, however, not curative, and may encourage the child to wet while asleep during the lifting.

NOTES:

URINE RETENTION AND FAILURE TO PASS URINE

The clinician overview

Retention of urine is a frequent presentation in adults but relatively infrequent in children. It constitutes a paediatric and genitourinary emergency. Retention of urine is defined as inability to void for over 12 hours, palpable distended bladder and greater than expected volume in the bladder in a child without known neurological abnormalities, voiding dysfunction, immobility or recent surgery. Presentation may be acute, requiring an immediate medical intervention such as catheterisation, or chronic. The normal neonates have 4–44 mL of urine in the bladder at birth. They are expected to pass urine within 48 hours of life (92% will do that by 24 hours), failure to void after 48 hours is abnormal and requires careful examination and investigation.

Possible diagnoses

INFANTS
Common
- Urethral valve obstruction
- Asphyxia/shock
- Dehydration
- Neurogenic bladder
- Acute renal failure

Rare
- Sepsis
- Acute tubular necrosis
- Acute genital herpes
- Congestive cardiac failure
- Bilateral renal agenesis
- Bilateral renal vein thrombosis
- Urethral stricture
- Ureterocele
- Disseminated intravascular coagulation (DIC)

CHILDREN

- Neurological abnormalities
- Severe voiding dysfunction
- Urinary tract infection (UTI)
- Constipation
- Drugs (anticholinergic, antidepressants)

- Local inflammation (e.g. balanoposthitis, urethritis)
- Dehydration
- Local inflammatory (balanitis, labial adhesions)
- Urethral calculus
- Foreign body inserted into the urethra
- Bladder neck obstruction
- DIC
- Ureterocele
- Tumour (e.g. rhabdomyosarcoma)

Differential diagnosis at a glance

	Neurological abnormalities	Severe voiding dysfunction	UTI	Constipation	Drugs
Abnormal urinalysis	Possible	Possible	Yes	Possible	No
Dysuria	No	Possible	Possible	Possible	Possible
Fever	No	No	Yes	No	No
Complete retention	Possible	No	No	Possible	Possible
Examination establishes the cause	Yes	No	No	Yes	No

Recommended investigations

*** Urinalysis: dipstick may show haematuria suggestive of urinary calculus or bladder tumour, or nitrite and leukocytes in favour of UTI.

*** U&E: high creatinine and urea suggest renal failure; high urea alone suggests dehydration.

*** Renal ultrasound scan: very helpful for constipation, dilated urethra, bladder and ureter.

TOP TIPS

- Over 90% of healthy newborns pass urine within 24 hours, the remaining within 48 hours.
- Posterior urethral valves are nowadays often discovered by antenatal ultrasound scan, which shows distended and thick-walled bladder.
- In normal children, having voiding intervals of more than 12 hours is unusual, therefore the above definition of retention.
- It is important to differentiate between anuria and retention. In the latter the bladder is usually full but empty with anuria. History, palpable bladder, abdominal X-ray and U&E differentiate between these conditions.
- Labial adhesions are a common condition (in up to 3% of girls) of urinary retention; topical oestrogen is indicated. Surgical intervention may be required.

Red flags

- ◪ For most cases of urinary retention, urgent urological referral is usually indicated.
- ◪ In suspected cases of urethral valve, do not catheterise the bladder before you contact a renal unit as this procedure may destroy the valve and the diagnosis can be missed.
- ◪ All cases of urine retention require admission for evaluation and management.
- ◪ Anticholinergic drugs used to stabilise the bladder for diurnal incontinence may cause retention, dry mouth and constipation. Parents should be warned about these possible side effects.
- ◪ A chronically distended bladder should not be drained fully by catheterisation – sudden decompression can cause haematuria and other renal complications.
- ◪ Massive haematuria can cause clots in the urethra causing bladder distention and retention.
- ◪ Urine retention may be the first sign of rhabdomyosarcoma; typical age for this is 2–4 years.

NOTES:

INDEX